NATIONAL ACADEMIES *Sciences Engineering Medicine*

NATIONAL ACADEMIES PRESS
Washington, DC

Visual Field Assessment and Disability Evaluation

Roger J. Lewis, Bernice X. Chu, Tina M. Winters, and Carol Mason Spicer, *Editors*

Committee on the Review of Standards for Visual Field Perimetry Devices and Their Use in Disability Evaluations

Board on Health Care Services

Health and Medicine Division

Consensus Study Report

NATIONAL ACADEMIES PRESS 500 Fifth Street, NW Washington, DC 20001

This activity was supported by Contract No. 28321323D00060012 between the National Academy of Sciences and U.S. Social Security Administration. Any opinions, findings, conclusions, or recommendations expressed in this publication do not necessarily reflect the views of any organization or agency that provided support for the project.

International Standard Book Number-13: 978-0-309-99252-7
Digital Object Identifier: https://doi.org/10.17226/29124

This publication is available from the National Academies Press, 500 Fifth Street, NW, Keck 360, Washington, DC 20001; (800) 624-6242; http://www.nap.nationalacademies.org.

The manufacturer's authorized representative in the European Union for product safety is Authorised Rep Compliance Ltd., Ground Floor, 71 Lower Baggot Street, Dublin D02 P593 Ireland; www.arccompliance.com

Copyright 2025 by the National Academy of Sciences. National Academies of Sciences, Engineering, and Medicine and National Academies Press and the graphical logos for each are all trademarks of the National Academy of Sciences. All rights reserved.

Printed in the United States of America.

Suggested citation: National Academies of Sciences, Engineering, and Medicine. 2025. *Visual field assessment and disability evaluation*. Washington, DC: National Academies Press. https://doi.org/10.17226/29124.

The **National Academy of Sciences** was established in 1863 by an Act of Congress, signed by President Lincoln, as a private, nongovernmental institution to advise the nation on issues related to science and technology. Members are elected by their peers for outstanding contributions to research. Dr. Marcia McNutt is president.

The **National Academy of Engineering** was established in 1964 under the charter of the National Academy of Sciences to bring the practices of engineering to advising the nation. Members are elected by their peers for extraordinary contributions to engineering. Dr. Tsu-Jae Liu is president.

The **National Academy of Medicine** (formerly the Institute of Medicine) was established in 1970 under the charter of the National Academy of Sciences to advise the nation on medical and health issues. Members are elected by their peers for distinguished contributions to medicine and health. Dr. Victor J. Dzau is president.

The three Academies work together as the **National Academies of Sciences, Engineering, and Medicine** to provide independent, objective analysis and advice to the nation and conduct other activities to solve complex problems and inform public policy decisions. The National Academies also encourage education and research, recognize outstanding contributions to knowledge, and increase public understanding in matters of science, engineering, and medicine.

Learn more about the National Academies of Sciences, Engineering, and Medicine at **www.nationalacademies.org**.

Consensus Study Reports published by the National Academies of Sciences, Engineering, and Medicine document the evidence-based consensus on the study's statement of task by an authoring committee of experts. Reports typically include findings, conclusions, and recommendations based on information gathered by the committee and the committee's deliberations. Each report has been subjected to a rigorous and independent peer-review process and it represents the position of the National Academies on the statement of task.

Proceedings published by the National Academies of Sciences, Engineering, and Medicine chronicle the presentations and discussions at a workshop, symposium, or other event convened by the National Academies. The statements and opinions contained in proceedings are those of the participants and are not endorsed by other participants, the planning committee, or the National Academies.

Rapid Expert Consultations published by the National Academies of Sciences, Engineering, and Medicine are authored by subject-matter experts on narrowly focused topics that can be supported by a body of evidence. The discussions contained in rapid expert consultations are considered those of the authors and do not contain policy recommendations. Rapid expert consultations are reviewed by the institution before release.

For information about other products and activities of the National Academies, please visit www.nationalacademies.org/about/whatwedo.

COMMITTEE ON THE REVIEW OF STANDARDS FOR VISUAL FIELD PERIMETRY DEVICES AND THEIR USE IN DISABILITY EVALUATIONS

ROGER J. LEWIS (*Chair*), David Geffen School of Medicine, University of California, Los Angeles
ROBERT CHUN, The State University of New York College of Optometry
STUART K. GARDINER, Devers Eye Institute
EVE J. HIGGINBOTHAM, Scheie Eye Institute, University of Pennsylvania
TIANJING LI, University of Colorado Anschutz Medical Campus
JULIUS T. OATTS, Children's Hospital of Philadelphia
ERIC L. SINGMAN, University of Maryland School of Medicine

Study Staff
BERNICE X. CHU, Senior Program Officer/Study Director
CAROL MASON SPICER, Senior Program Officer
TINA M. WINTERS, Program Officer
LYLE CARRERA, Research Associate
CHIDINMA CHUKWURAH, Senior Program Assistant
JOSEPH GOODMAN, Senior Program Assistant
SHARYL NASS, Senior Board Director, Board on Health Care Services

Reviewers

This Consensus Study Report was reviewed in draft form by individuals chosen for their diverse perspectives and technical expertise. The purpose of this independent review is to provide candid and critical comments that will assist the National Academies of Sciences, Engineering, and Medicine in making each published report as sound as possible and to ensure that it meets the institutional standards for quality, objectivity, evidence, and responsiveness to the study charge. The review comments and draft manuscript remain confidential to protect the integrity of the deliberative process.

We thank the following individuals for their review of this report:

AVA BITTNER, University of California, Los Angeles
CLAUDE DESPLAN, New York University
JOSHUA R. EHRLICH, University of Michigan
HOWARD H. GOLDMAN, University of Maryland
GENA HEIDARY, Boston Children's Hospital, Harvard Medical School
MICHAEL KALLONIATIS, University of Houston
ALISON LIU, University of Colorado Anschutz Medical Campus
J. JASON McANANY, University of Illinois at Chicago
PRADEEP RAMULU, Johns Hopkins University

Although the reviewers listed above provided many constructive comments and suggestions, they were not asked to endorse the conclusions or recommendations of this report, nor did they see the final draft before its release. The review of this report was overseen by **ROBERT S. LAWRENCE,** Bloomberg School of Public Health, Johns Hopkins University, and **THOMAS D. ALBRIGHT,** Salk Institute for Biological Studies. They were responsible for making certain that an independent examination of this report was carried out in accordance with the standards of the National Academies and that all review comments were carefully considered. Responsibility for the final content rests entirely with the authoring committee and the National Academies.

Contents

PREFACE   xiii

ACRONYMS AND ABBREVIATIONS   xvii

SUMMARY   1
    Context for This Study, 1
    Study Charge and Scope, 3
    Study Approach, 4
    The Committee's Conclusions, 5

1 INTRODUCTION   17
    Study Charge and Scope, 18
    Prevalence of Visual Field Loss and Its Impact
       on Quality of Life, 19
    SSA's Disability Evaluation Process, 24
    SSA's Current Standards for Measuring Visual Fields, 25
    Study Approach, 29
    Organization of the Report, 30
    References, 31

2 HOW OTHER SELECTED FEDERAL AGENCIES ASSESS
    IMPAIRMENT DUE TO VISUAL FIELD LOSS   37
    Disability Benefits, 38
    Employment Qualifications, 40

Functional Criteria, 43
Summary and Conclusion, 45
References, 46

3 **CURRENT AND EMERGING PRACTICE IN VISUAL FIELD TESTING**   49
Fundamentals of Perimetry, 51
Current Practice in Perimetry Assessment, 62
Variability and Challenges in the Clinical Assessment of Visual Fields, 67
Recent Changes in Practice, 71
Summary and Conclusions, 77
References, 79

4 **EVALUATING NEW PERIMETRY TECHNIQUES**   83
Design of Studies for Assessing Diagnostic Test Accuracy, 83
Performance Considerations for Evaluating New Perimetry Techniques, 87
Quantity and Characteristics of Validation Studies Needed to Find a Perimeter Acceptable, 94
Summary and Conclusions, 94
References, 96

5 **SPECIAL TOPICS**   99
Optical Projection Versus Screen-Based Stimuli, 100
Frequency Doubling Technology, 104
Semiautomated Kinetic Perimetry, 109
Alternatives to Kinetic Perimetry for Testing Visual Field Efficiency, 116
Pediatric Considerations, 121
Summary, 123
References, 124

APPENDIXES

Appendix A	Public Meeting Agendas	131
Appendix B	Glossary	133
Appendix C	Biographical Sketches of Committee Members	139

Boxes, Figures, and Tables

BOXES

S-1 Definitions of Key Terms Used in This Report, 2
S-2 Statement of Task, 4

1-1 Statement of Task, 18
1-2 Definitions of Key Terms Used in This Report, 20

3-1 Types of Visual Field Losses, 50

FIGURES

1-1 Diagram of the eight principal meridians for each eye, 28

3-1 Simulation of selected types of visual field losses, 50
3-2 Normal hill of vision for a right eye, 51
3-3 The human visual pathway, 53
3-4 Static automated threshold perimetry testing experience, 54
3-5 Goldmann stimulus sizes, 55
3-6 Humphrey visual field printout, 57
3-7 Example of Goldmann visual field plot, 60
3-8 Examples of testing patterns (right eye), 66
3-9 imo head-mounted automated perimeter, 72
3-10 Example of a Gabor patch, 74

5-1 Visual characteristics of stimuli used in second-generation frequency doubling technology (FDT2) and static automated threshold perimetry (SAP), 105
5-2 Visual field from static automated threshold perimetry (SAP) and frequency doubling technology (FDT), 107
5-3 Diagram of the eight principal meridians for each eye, 112

TABLES

1-1 Summary of Pathways to Meeting the Social Security Administration's Listing Criteria for Visual Disorders, 26

3-1 Field Testing Instruments, Testing Strategies, Testing Patterns, and Testing Algorithms, 63

4-1 Reference Standards Used in Perimetry Validation Studies, 85

5-1 Summary of Stimuli in Standard and Selected Novel Perimeters, 101
5-2 Diagnostic Agreement Between Octopus Semiautomated Kinetic Perimetry and Humphrey Field Analyzer Static Automated Perimetry, 113

ANNEX TABLE

Annex Table 1-1 Selected Excerpts Relevant to Visual Field Testing from Social Security Administration Documents, 33

Preface

It is projected that the number of individuals who will become visually impaired will double by the year 2050, affecting nearly 7 million individuals within the United States. Among these affected individuals will be a significant proportion of adults who rely on their vision to support themselves and their families. Visual field loss, even to a degree that fails to meet the criteria for statutory blindness, can have profound impacts on virtually all aspects of life, including the ability to be gainfully employed; for many adults the ability to maintain normal or nearly normal visual function is critical for performing the vast majority of tasks associated with their employment. As noted in the 2016 National Academies of Sciences, Engineering, and Medicine report entitled *Making Eye Health a Population Health Imperative*, the impact of visual impairment is increased when it is coupled with other chronic conditions such as depression, stroke, and cardiac conditions, which plague many working adults. Similarly, for children, the ability to see is critical for their everyday activities, including participation in educational and social activities. It has been estimated that as many as 5 percent of preschool aged children suffer from visual impairment. Accordingly, the Social Security Administration (SSA) has established standards for defining disabling, uncorrectable visual field loss, relative to that required for gainful activity in adults, or for participation in age-appropriate activities in children.

The assessment of visual function is key in identifying and assessing limitations in an individual's ability to complete tasks that require unimpaired vision. While the measure of correctable visual acuity satisfies the question of clarity of vision, the measure of visual field provides additional information regarding the boundaries of an individual's entire visual landscape. The importance of the visual field is underscored by the definition of statutory blindness, which can be met by a sufficiently constricted field of vision, even when visual acuity is normal. The assessment of one's visual field, as measured using perimetric testing, is a core metric to determine one's level of visual impairment.

There are important variations in the availability and use of tests to assess visual field loss across populations and geographic locations. Progress in the field of perimetry, defined as the measurement of the ability to perceive contrasting stimuli across specific locations of the visual field, holds out the promise to improve the availability of testing to identify applicants for disability benefits who meet SSA criteria based on visual field loss. Because visual field loss can take many different forms, e.g., scotoma or blind spots, decreased sensitivity to light in the periphery or in specific areas of the visual field, SSA standards include multiple potential routes to qualification for benefits, with different standards being most applicable to different patterns of visual field loss. Moreover, new technology provides more effective strategies for determining visual field defects that meet SSA requirements. Barriers to the assessment of visual field loss relative to SSA disability standards could be lowered if acceptable testing could be conducted in a wider variety of settings, and with a wider range of providers, perimetry techniques, and devices. Thus, SSA requested that an ad hoc committee of the National Academy of Sciences, Engineering, and Medicine be convened to address specific questions regarding the use of perimetry, including the use of newer devices and technologies, in assessing qualification for SSA disability benefits based on visual field loss.

On behalf of the entire committee, I would like to extend my sincere thanks to the many individuals who shared their time and expertise to support and inform our work and deliberations. The study was sponsored by SSA, and I thank Vincent Nibali and Michael Goldstein for their guidance and support. I also acknowledge Vincent Nibali at SSA for verifying the accuracy of relevant technical content pertaining to the disability determination process. The committee also benefited greatly from discussions with individuals who participated in the committee's open sessions: Sylvia Groth, Chris Johnson, Yao Liu, Paula Anne Newman-Casey, George Spaeth, and Varshini Varadaraj, as well as the individuals who shared their experiences with accessing care for visual field impairments and applying for disability: LaQuilla Harris, Christopher Hord, and Zelda Kitchens.

I thank all members of the committee for generously contributing their time and expertise to this task, for the benefit of those living with visual impairment. I also thank the reviewers of this report for their invaluable feedback on an earlier draft and the monitor and coordinator who oversaw the report review, as well as committee member Eve J. Higginbotham for help with this preface.

Also on behalf of the committee, I would like to acknowledge the many staff within the Health and Medicine Division (HMD) who provided support in various ways to this project, including Bernice Chu (study director), Carol Mason Spicer (senior program officer), Tina Winters (program officer [Board on Cognitive and Behavioral Sciences, Division of Behavioral and Social Sciences and Education]), Lyle Carrera (research associate), Violet Bishop (research associate), Chidinma Chukwurah (senior program assistant), and Joseph Goodman (senior program assistant). I also extend my appreciation to Sharyl Nass, senior board director, Board on Health Care Services, who oversaw the project. Greysi Patton (finance business partner), Julie Wiltshire (senior finance business partner), and Ron Brown (deputy director, HMD program finance) oversaw finances for the project, and the report review, production, and communications staff all provided valuable guidance to ensure the success of the final product. Rona Briere, Allison Boman, and Danielle Nasenbeny provided superb editorial guidance in preparing the final report. Crystal Mitchell (University of Maryland Ophthalmology) lent her time and expertise to ensure the report included high-quality perimetry testing images.

Roger J. Lewis, *Chair*
Committee on the Review of Standards for
Visual Field Perimetry Devices and Their Use in Disability Evaluations

Acronyms and Abbreviations

ADA	Americans with Disabilities Act
AIZE	Ambient Interactive ZEST
AMA	American Medical Association
asb	apostilb
cd	candela
dB	decibel
DCM	*Disability Claims Manual*
EEOC	Equal Employment Opportunity Commission
FAA	Federal Aviation Administration
FDA	Food and Drug Administration
FDP	frequency doubling perimetry
FDT	frequency doubling technology
FDT1	first-generation frequency doubling technology
FDT2	second-generation frequency doubling technology
FERS	Federal Employees Retirement System
FMCSA	Federal Motor Carrier Safety Administration
FRA	Federal Railroad Administration
HFA	Humphrey Field Analyzer
HRQoL	health-related quality of life
Hz	hertz

IDEA	Individuals with Disabilities Education Act
LCD	liquid-crystal display
LED	light-emitting diode
MD	mean deviation
M-pathway	magnocellular pathway
NHANES	National Health and Nutrition Examination Survey
OLED	organic light-emitting diode
OSEP	Office of Special Education Programs (Department of Education)
OWCP	Office of Workers' Compensation Programs (Department of Labor)
P-pathway	parvocellular pathway
PSD	pattern standard deviation
QUADAS-2	Quality Assessment of Diagnostic Accuracy Studies 2
RRB	Railroad Retirement Board
SAP	static automated threshold perimetry
SITA	Swedish Interactive Thresholding Algorithm
SSA	Social Security Administration
SSDI	Social Security Disability Insurance
SSI	Supplemental Security Income
SVOP	saccadic vector optokinetic perimetry
SWAP	short-wavelength automated perimetry
TOP	tendency-oriented perimetry
U.S.	United States
USPSTF	United States Preventive Services Task Force
VAE	visual acuity efficiency
VAI	visual acuity impairment value
VFE	visual field efficiency
VFI	visual field impairment value or visual field index
VR	virtual reality
ZEST	Zippy Estimation by Sequential Testing

Summary[1]

Visual field impairment is associated with a number of conditions, including glaucoma, optic neuropathies, and disorders affecting the retina and visual pathways. Significant loss of visual field impacts quality of life and can result in varying degrees of disability. This is particularly true with respect to a person's daily functioning, including the ability to work and participate in school; social engagement; and emotional well-being. Individuals with moderate to severe visual field loss may have difficulty performing routine tasks such as reading, driving, and navigating different environments, which leads in turn to greater reliance on others and reduced independence. Visual field loss also limits the ability to engage in social activities, thereby reducing overall social participation and contributing to feelings of isolation. The degree of impact varies depending on the severity of the loss, with more profound loss leading to greater disability and poorer quality of life.

CONTEXT FOR THIS STUDY

Perimetry, also known as visual field testing, is an essential tool for assessing ophthalmic conditions that can result in visual field loss. Perimetry techniques consist of a combination of hardware, stimuli, testing patterns, and algorithms. These techniques form the complex and highly technical context for the present study. (See Box S-1 for definitions of the key technical terms used in this report.)

---

[1] This summary does not include references. Citations to support the discussion and conclusions herein are provided in the main text.

> **BOX S-1**
> **Definitions of Key Terms Used in This Report**
>
> **Visual field** is the total area of space a person can see when the eyes are focused on a central point.
>
> **Visual field meridians** refer to imaginary lines radiating from a center point that divide the visual field into equal sections, like pieces of a pie.
>
> **Visual perimeter device (perimeter)** is a machine used to measure visual fields.
>
> **Visual perimetry** is the systematic measurement of visual fields.
>
> **Automated perimetry** refers to automated presentation of the test stimulus and recording of patient responses.
>
> **Static perimetry** refers to stationary stimuli presented at defined points in the visual field. Locations at which the stimulus is seen and not seen are recorded.
>
> **Kinetic perimetry** uses a moving stimulus that is generally moved from a nonseeing area to seeing area in a systematic way to map the central and peripheral visual field boundaries, in addition to any scotomas, including blind spots. This movement can be automated, semiautomated, or manual.
>
> **Static automated threshold perimetry**[a] refers to the projection of a white stimulus onto a white background to determine the probable threshold at chosen locations in the visual field. Blue on yellow static automated threshold perimetry is also available.
>
> **Automated kinetic perimetry**[b] uses a moving stimulus of a selected size and intensity, with the speed and direction of the stimulus being automated.

It is in this context that the Social Security Administration (SSA) must determine whether applicants with visual field loss qualify for benefits under one of the agency's disability programs. As part of its disability determination process, SSA considers whether an applicant would qualify for disability benefits on the basis of criteria specified in its Listing of Impairments—specifically those in the Special Senses and Speech Listings for both adults and children, which include criteria requiring the use of specific types of perimetry and perimeters. For individuals for whom the required tests are not accessible, it may be difficult or even impossible to be approved for disability benefits.

Optical projection consists of projecting a light stimulus onto a background to present it to the patient's eye in order to map the visual field.

Frequency doubling technology, used in some perimeters, is based on a flicker illusion, which essentially creates an image that appears double its actual spatial frequency. The stimulus does not move across the field, and the flickering is a proxy for the stimulus intensity used in either static or kinetic perimetry.

Visual acuity is a measure of the sharpness or clarity of vision at a given distance.

Visual field efficiency (SSA definition) is expressed as a percentage corresponding to the visual field in the better eye, calculated by adding the number of degrees seen along the eight principal meridians found on a visual field chart and dividing by 5.

Mean deviation is the average difference in visual field sensitivity across all measured locations compared with a normal, age-matched reference field.

Statutory blindness refers to blindness as defined in the Social Security Act: (1) "central visual acuity of 20/200 or less in the better eye with the use of a correcting lens" or (2) "an eye that has a visual field limitation such that the widest diameter of the visual field subtends an angle no greater than 20 degrees" (Social Security Act, sections 216[i][1]; 1614[a][2]).

---

[a] Multiple terms are used to refer to the same technology. This report preferentially uses the term *static automated threshold perimetry* to distinguish it from other types of perimetry (e.g., kinetic, manual, suprathreshold).

[b] Although *automated (or automatic) kinetic perimetry* is typically used in the literature, this report preferentially uses the term *semiautomated kinetic perimetry* to be more precise about the role of the technician in administering the test.

STUDY CHARGE AND SCOPE

In August 2024, SSA requested that the Health and Medicine Division of the National Academies of Sciences, Engineering, and Medicine convene an ad hoc committee of relevant experts[2] to review the latest published research and science on visual perimetry devices. The committee

---

[2] The committee included experts in ophthalmology (adult and pediatric), neuro-ophthalmology, optometry, optical science, internal medicine, measurement validation, and SSA disability policy.

> **BOX S-2**
> **Statement of Task**
>
> The task order objectives for the ad hoc committee of the National Academies of Sciences, Engineering, and Medicine are to review the latest published research and science and produce a report addressing best practices and known limitations in the use of visual perimeter devices to measure visual field loss in connection with disability evaluations, including
>
> 1. Describing the current practice landscape for the measurement of visual field impairment with visual perimeter devices, and recent changes or challenges in the provision of such care; and
> 2. Answering the following questions based on published evidence (to the extent possible) and professional judgment (where published evidence is lacking):
>   a. Is optical projection of the testing stimuli still a necessity to achieve valid and reliable results from a perimeter? How does the eye respond differently to projected stimulus vs. other types (e.g., LCD screens)?
>   b. Do perimeters using frequency doubling technology produce substantially similar results to traditional perimeters and what differences are there?

was charged with producing a report addressing best practices and known limitations in the use of visual perimeter devices to measure visual field loss in connection with SSA's disability evaluations. This review was to include identifying the latest standards of care regarding measurement of an individual's visual fields. The committee also was asked to review the devices, techniques, and standards used by other federal agencies to make determinations of statutory blindness based on visual field loss. The committee's work was to be based on published evidence (to the extent possible) and professional judgment (where such evidence is lacking). Box S-2 contains the committee's full statement of task. SSA requested that the committee's report include conclusions, but not recommendations.

STUDY APPROACH

The committee met four times to discuss the questions posed in the statement of task and held a public information-gathering session to hear from invited speakers about disparities and opportunities in access to vision testing, lived experiences with visual impairment and applying for

c. Is automatic kinetic perimetry a valid and reliable method of measuring visual field loss? What are the necessary device specifications and testing circumstances for automatic kinetic perimetry to produce valid and reliable visual field testing?
d. What are the most widely acceptable and commonly used alternatives to kinetic perimetry, both manual and automated, for the measurement of visual field efficiency? What impacts do such alternative methods have on the validity and reliability of testing results?
e. From a medical and practical perspective, is it still necessary for SSA to require three published clinical validation studies to find a perimeter acceptable or could fewer studies potentially show validity with similar reliability? If fewer validation studies could be acceptable, would there be higher requirements on the design or execution of those studies?
f. What devices, techniques, and standards are other federal agencies using to make statutory blindness determinations based on visual field loss?

The report will include findings and conclusions but not recommendations.

SSA disability benefits, and emerging technologies in visual field testing. These speakers informed the committee's understanding of challenges in providing care for visual field impairment and how such impairment can affect employment, day-to-day life, and general well-being.

After discussing each item in the statement of task, the committee reached consensus on its conclusions, which reflect the published evidence and the committee members' professional judgment where published evidence is lacking. Additionally, National Academies staff conducted a broad scoping search of perimetry validation studies published since 2002. This review supported the committee's discussion of the essential elements of an effective perimetry validation study while helping to ensure that the standards discussed were achievable.

THE COMMITTEE'S CONCLUSIONS

The committee formulated 17 conclusions about visual field testing in the following areas: (1) visual field testing in federal agencies, (2) current and emerging practice in visual field testing, (3) evaluating new perimetry techniques, and (4) special topics in visual field testing. (Note that the numbering of the conclusions here is the same as that in the report chapters [e.g., Conclusion 2-1 is found in Chapter 2 of the report]).

Visual Field Testing in Federal Agencies

As mentioned, SSA specifies requirements for visual field testing to inform its disability determinations. These requirements clarify when and how different methods, such as static automated threshold perimetry and manual or semiautomated kinetic perimetry, are to be used, ensuring that test results align with SSA's standards. Like SSA, many other government agencies have their own definitions of disability and visual impairment and their accepted methods for assessing visual field loss. Those assessments are used to determine eligibility for disability benefits, eligibility for other disability-related programs, or qualification for certain jobs. Most go beyond the federal definition of statutory blindness, which requires that the widest diameter of a person's visual field be 20 degrees or less. Some agencies, like SSA, use statutory blindness as one of several medical criteria for a person to qualify as disabled. Others adopt a functional definition of visual impairment that is based on potential obstacles to engaging in relevant daily tasks. Most, however, set a specific visual field size that examinees must meet or not meet. The preferred perimeters and measurement techniques also differ among agencies, with some permitting a broader selection than others.

Some agencies use visual field assessment to determine eligibility for employment in jobs requiring good vision. The varying requirements in occupationally based visual assessment suggest that the bar for meaningful visual impairment is vocation specific. Other federal programs define visual impairment or disability based on functional criteria rather than specific diagnostic measures, emphasizing the impact on activities such as education or daily living. Federal programs designed to promote equality of access to, for example, education similarly define eligibility using functional criteria, such as a person's inability to access standard educational materials, verified by qualified experts. This approach highlights the emphasis on functional impact over the type of objective medical criteria found in federal disability evaluations.

Based on its review of the literature, the committee reached the following conclusion:

Conclusion 2.1: Different federal government agencies have their own definitions of disability and visual impairment and their accepted methods for assessing visual field loss for a variety of purposes, including determining eligibility for disability benefits, eligibility for other disability-related programs, or qualification for certain jobs.

Current and Emerging Practice in Visual Field Testing

Perimetry is an essential diagnostic tool for assessing a variety of ophthalmic conditions. As noted previously, perimetry techniques consist of a combination of hardware, stimuli (e.g., luminance, size), testing patterns, and algorithms. Static automated threshold perimetry measures the sensitivity of an individual's visual fields at specific test locations and has the capability to compare the findings with a normal database of previously tested patients. Specific programs can be used to tailor the test to focus on the visual field loss of the patient. Manual or semiautomated kinetic perimetry may also be used by eye care providers to assess visual fields. However, semiautomated techniques are used more commonly than manual ones because of the need for trained personnel to conduct the latter and because of the ability to standardize testing conditions with the former.

Recent changes in practice include newer algorithms that reduce the number of stimuli presented to the patient and quickly learn which additional points should be tested based on previous responses. The shorter testing times made possible by these algorithms decrease reliability, although not significantly. Testing algorithms are not mentioned in the SSA listings, but they are important, as test performance is algorithm specific. Moreover, as visual field loss worsens, variability in performance increases. In other words, for individuals who are sufficiently impaired to be categorized as disabled, variability in test results will increase. Given the learning curve in visual field testing, conducting multiple tests might improve the accuracy of the results. It is unclear how many visual field tests might be required to achieve optimum accuracy, but administering a minimum of two tests may improve results, particularly in patients naïve to visual field tests.

SSA's listing criteria for assessing mean deviation requires a Humphrey Field Analyzer 30-2 test result. The committee notes, however, that the 30-2 testing pattern is used less often now in routine practice and that the 30-2 and 24-2 test patterns are functionally equivalent in many instances. Manual and semiautomated kinetic perimetry also are not needed except for special circumstances, such as for SSA's calculation of visual field efficiency.

Based on its review of the literature, the committee reached the following conclusions:

Conclusion 3.1: Measurement of visual field impairment involves components beyond the hardware or visual perimetry device, including stimuli, testing patterns, and algorithms. All components are important to consider when evaluating the validity of visual field assessment.

Conclusion 3.2: Because variability in the results of visual field assessment increases as the severity of visual field impairment increases, and given the learning curve in visual field testing, more than one visual field test may be needed to characterize an individual's visual field impairment accurately.

Conclusion 3.3: The Social Security Administration's listing criteria for assessing mean deviation require a Humphrey Field Analyzer 30-2 test result, but this testing pattern is used less often now in routine practice. In many instances, however, the 24-2 testing pattern is functionally equivalent to the 30-2 testing pattern and may be sufficient for assessing mean deviation.

Perimetry outcomes can vary as a result of patient-related factors, differences in perimeters and how perimetry is performed, and systems-level factors. Patient-related factors include whether a patient possesses the mental and physical capacity to participate in the testing, the patient's previous experience with perimetric testing, their use of alcohol and medications that may suppress the central nervous system, the presence of diseases such as diabetes or arthritis, the patient's level of fatigue, and ocular conditions that may affect the ability to fixate. Perimetry results can also vary depending on choices made by examiners, including the type of perimeter used, the order in which the left and right eyes are tested, and whether patients are supervised and well positioned during the testing. With respect to systems-level factors, visual field testing using traditional perimeters such as the Humphrey Field Analyzer (static automated) and Octopus (semiautomated kinetic) requires oversight by experienced technicians, creating challenges for individuals with limited access to appropriately trained eye care providers. Expanding vision care to settings such as primary care, health clinics, and federally qualified health centers can improve access. Emerging cost-effective technologies, such as virtual reality headsets and tablet- and desktop-based systems, also show promise for improving accessibility. Virtual reality headsets offer high-resolution stimuli and built-in eye tracking, which can provide an accurate measure of fixation stability and thus improve test reliability. Tablets and desktop systems leverage widely available devices to facilitate home testing, but they face challenges that can impact reliability, such as uncontrolled lighting, inconsistent viewing angles, and reduced standardization of test conditions.

Based on its review of the literature, the committee reached the following conclusion:

Conclusion 3.4: Visual field testing with traditional perimeters such as the Humphrey Field Analyzer and Octopus requires oversight by experienced technicians who may be in limited supply, creating challenges for some populations with limited access to care. Emerging cost-effective technologies, such as virtual reality headsets and tablet- and desktop-based systems, show promise for improving accessibility. With proper design and implementation, these tools may significantly expand access to visual field testing while maintaining reliability and validity, assuming studies demonstrate the ability to provide accurate, reproducible results even in an unsupervised setting and their suitability for determining SSA disability in the target population.

Evaluating New Perimetry Techniques

Validating a new perimetry technique requires a thorough assessment of its validity, reliability indices, and reproducibility, all aligned with its intended use in SSA disability determination. The ideal study assessing a new perimetry technique is designed so that it directly evaluates the technique's intended use and target population—for this report, specifically to determine whether an individual meets the criteria for visual field loss in connection with SSA disability determination. Given that the committee's review of the literature revealed no studies that directly examined a perimetry technique for this specific purpose, one could use correlation between the results obtained with a new technique and those obtained with a reference standard perimeter in eyes with moderate and/or severe functional loss as a proxy. As reference standards are typically the current "gold standard," comparing new perimeters to the Humphrey Field Analyzer using a size III stimulus may generate useful evidence.

Determination of the acceptability of a perimetry technique needs to focus on its specific combination of testing algorithm, stimuli, and device rather than being based solely on the device itself. Also essential is to take the scope of evidence into account, including data from diverse populations and real-world settings, to ensure that the technique performs effectively across patients with various underlying clinical conditions. Risk of bias assessment is also important.

Based on its review of the literature and the committee's expert assessment, the committee reached the following conclusions:

Conclusion 4.1: When assessing the acceptability of a technique for visual field assessment, the quality, relevance, and totality of the evidence are more important than the number of published studies available.

Conclusion 4.2: Sensitivity (in the sense of a test's ability to identify correctly those with a qualifying disability) and specificity (a test's capacity to identify correctly those without a qualifying disability) are important metrics for assessing a test's internal validity. Both specificity and sensitivity need to be measured with sufficient precision to permit confident evaluation against the SSA criteria.

Many perimeters report statistics such as fixation losses and false-positive and false-negative results. While these reliability indices provide useful information about how a perimetry test was conducted, it is not always appropriate to treat them as fixed binary cutoffs. Instead, it is important to examine a test result that appears to have poor reliability to determine why poor reliability indices were measured and whether there is sufficient information for the assessment of disability.

Based on its review of the literature, the committee reached the following conclusion:

Conclusion 4.3: Test results that appear to have poor reliability indices need to be examined to determine whether the results may still be useful for identifying deficits that qualify for disability benefits by providing sufficient information for the determination of disability.

With intensities above 15–20 decibels (dB) on a Humphrey Field Analyzer perimeter or the equivalent on other instruments, the probability of an examinee responding to the stimulus plateaus. Therefore, further increases in brightness (decrease in dBs) have minimal impact on detectability, hindering accurate measurement of severe field loss. Variability in results may also arise from different levels of contrast. Research has shown that testing with contrasts greater than 15–20 dB does not enhance the ability to detect disease progression and can be excluded without loss of information.

Based on its review of the literature and the committee's expert assessment, the committee reached the following conclusion:

Conclusion 4.4: Although SSA's current criteria for visual disability require the ability to detect a stimulus corresponding to 10-dB contrast on a Humphrey Field Analyzer perimeter, it is likely that equivalent results can be achieved using a stimulus corresponding to a 15-dB contrast.

Special Topics in Visual Field Testing

Optical Projection Versus Screen-Based Stimuli

A strong and growing body of literature suggests the acceptable clinical performance of perimeters that do not use optical stimulus projection. While theoretically, the perception of projected and nonprojected stimuli that are otherwise similar should be the same, scientific evidence specifically evaluating the consistency of test results using different types of stimuli is limited.

Screen-based perimeters may become more acceptable and reliable for the average patient, as they are both cheaper than traditional perimeters and based on common consumer electronics. Virtual reality perimeters, in particular, may be able to include eye tracking and adjust for fixation, which would make them far more reliable than traditional techniques. As these technologies develop, allowing their use for SSA disability determination would make perimetry easier, more available, and less costly for more people.

At present, however, these new technologies come with substantial uncertainties in performance. Luminance varies significantly among different screen-based perimeters, and stimuli may not be exactly the same as in traditional perimeters because of limitations in modern screen-based technology. Many screen-based perimeters are also not able to achieve the range of luminance (especially at the dim end) that is achieved in table-top perimeters.

Device manufacturers can mitigate these challenges in a variety of ways, such as by modifying the stimulus intensity, size, and duration. Different test patterns may also be feasible in the future. In theory, variations in these design factors could result in stimuli functionally equivalent to those presented by traditional perimeters. To best validate these perimeters for use in SSA disability determination, their performance in relevant classification tasks should be compared with that of currently accepted projection-based methods.

Based on its review of this evidence and the committee's expert assessment, the committee reached the following conclusions:

Conclusion 5.1: The technology used to present stimuli and backgrounds during perimetry, such as optical projection or video screens, is unlikely to have a substantial effect on visual perception or test results. However, because perimeters using nonprojected visuals have been developed only relatively recently, evaluation studies of such perimeters will be most useful if they robustly report specific testing parameters and the technical details of the device.

Conclusion 5.2: The suitability of novel perimeters for SSA's use in disability determination is affected by their performance relative to that of current methods; comparative validation studies, ideally using SSA-relevant classification tasks, will therefore be the best way to assess suitability.

Frequency Doubling Technology

Frequency doubling technology (FDT) is a specialized visual field–testing method that uses high-frequency flickering stimuli to assess the integrity of the visual field. It is typically used as a screening test, especially for early or mild visual field impairment caused by glaucoma. Perimeters using FDT tend to be less expensive and easier to use than static automated threshold perimeters for both clinicians and examinees, and they tend to yield similar results in patients with early or mild glaucomatous impairment. Although results across studies regarding its sensitivity, specificity, and agreement of its results with those of static automated threshold perimetry are mixed, the differences are greatest in cases of severe impairment. FDT also gives very poor results in patients with cataracts, making it difficult to interpret results and potentially leading to results that may not reflect a true defect. Ultimately, more studies aimed at validating the use of FDT for diagnostic tasks such as those performed by SSA will be the most useful research.

Based on its review of the literature and the committee's expert assessment, the committee reached the following conclusions:

Conclusion 5.3: Second-generation frequency doubling technology (FDT2) devices have demonstrated similarity to traditional perimeters in the measurement of visual field contrast sensitivity; however, most studies thus far have been conducted in individuals with mild to moderate visual impairment. Additional studies are needed to determine the suitability of these devices for assessing visual function in individuals with severe visual impairment.

Conclusion 5.4: Because of its portability and lower cost, frequency doubling technology is likely to be particularly useful in settings where patients have limited access to static automated threshold perimetry and other traditional perimeters.

Semiautomated Kinetic Perimetry

Semiautomated kinetic perimetry can be used to determine disability as defined by SSA; it can identify peripheral visual defects outside the central 30 degrees, a requirement for calculating visual field efficiency as defined by SSA. In addition, semiautomated kinetic perimetry adds value over manual kinetic perimetry because it requires less of a learning curve and operators require less technical expertise and training.

At the same time, kinetic perimetry (either manual or semiautomated) has limitations. First, the results of kinetic perimetry tend to be less concordant with those of static automated threshold perimetry methods when used to assess the central visual field; therefore, kinetic perimetry is more often used at the periphery. Moreover, to realize the full potential of kinetic perimetry for full-field and peripheral visual field assessment, an examiner needs experience and training beyond that required by static perimetry. A skilled technician can monitor for fixation loss, check for false negatives or positives, and plot more complicated scotomas. In particular, ineffective monitoring of fixation can lead to overestimation of visual field performance. As a result, static automated threshold perimetry may be preferred if the patient presents with generalized constriction of the visual field and neither peripheral "islands of vision" nor ring scotomas are likely. Static automated threshold perimetry uses standardized algorithms to plot threshold contrast sensitivities automatically within the central 48–60 degrees of the visual field.

In addition, acquiring an Octopus perimeter (the most common platform capable of performing semiautomated kinetic testing) may be prohibitively expensive, and even where these devices are available, technicians adequately trained to use them may not be available. If Octopus perimeters were the only machines SSA considered acceptable for employing semiautomated kinetic strategies, then given the associated cost and training constraints, permitting semiautomated kinetic perimetry might yield only modest improvements in the availability of visual field testing. On the other hand, some clinics may have only an Octopus or other semiautomated kinetic perimeter, or an individual clinician may prefer using this form of perimetry.

Based on its review of the literature, the committee reached the following conclusion:

Conclusion 5.5: When administered by a skilled technician, semiautomated kinetic perimetry has sufficient accuracy in quantifying visual field efficiency for use by SSA in disability determinations.

Alternatives to Kinetic Perimetry for Visual Field Efficiency

While static automated threshold perimetry is available to measure peripheral vision, it may not suffice for measuring the full extent of the visual field, as required by SSA for the calculation of visual field efficiency. For most people seeking disability benefits, however, this limitation does not make much of a difference; a person found to qualify for disability benefits using a 60-degree perimeter likely would have a sufficiently constrained visual field to qualify and would not need additional testing with a perimeter to test further boundaries. Furthermore, static automated threshold perimetry is currently far more commonly available than semiautomated kinetic perimetry, and it can be performed with more consistency and less examiner bias than manual kinetic perimetry.

Allowing the use of static automated threshold perimetry for assessing visual field efficiency may yield uncertain or inadequate results in some scenarios. Since all of the current commercially available instruments and testing methods have their own limitations with respect to the clinical information they provide, multiple tests with the same method or an array of methods may be required to provide a better understanding of the extent of visual field loss. For example, kinetic perimetry could be used to measure at the peripheral field, while static automated threshold perimetry could be used centrally.

Although static automated threshold perimetry is not a "one-to-one" substitution for kinetic perimetry, it usually can provide the data required to calculate visual field efficiency. However, there may be rare exceptions. It is theoretically possible that a ring scotoma, such as those seen in retinitis pigmentosa, could leave the entire visual field past 60 degrees unaffected. Using static automated threshold perimetry for measurement of visual field efficiency in such a person could yield a technical "false positive" that would result in approving that person for disability benefits. However, the committee believes that the overall disability experienced by such an individual with significant ring scotomas or midperipheral visual field loss is otherwise likely to provide sufficient evidence to result in a disability determination.

Use of a larger stimulus size can increase the reliability of static automated threshold perimetry at the periphery. The currently mandated size III Goldmann stimulus has resulted in increased intertest variability and lower sensitivity, especially at the periphery. A size V stimulus would be more feasible and reliable if static automated threshold perimetry were to be used to assess visual field efficiency.

Based on its review of the literature, the committee reached the following conclusions:

> Conclusion 5.6: Despite the limitations of static automated threshold perimetry (SAP) in measuring peripheral field loss, this method can usually provide the data necessary to calculate the visual field efficiency of an applicant for SSA disability benefits.

- *Visual field efficiencies calculated using SAP will generally be diagnostically equivalent to those calculated using currently approved manual (Goldmann) kinetic or semiautomated kinetic perimetry; applicants who qualify for benefits using one will almost always qualify using the other.*
- *Even in exceedingly rare scenarios in which a person qualifies for disability benefits based on SAP assessment of visual field efficiency whereas in fact, the regions of the peripheral visual field outside the region mapped by SAP have preserved vision to a degree that the true visual field efficiency would not meet SSA requirements, the overall disability experienced by the applicant is likely to provide sufficient evidence to result in a disability determination.*

Conclusion 5.7: The use of larger stimuli, further diagnostic tests, and other clinical data can improve the diagnostic reliability of static automated threshold perimetry for the calculation of visual field efficiency.

Pediatric Considerations

Given the practical considerations involved in evaluating visual field in children across a range of ages and developmental statuses, there is particular value in increased flexibility in perimetry requirements for the pediatric population. Additionally, newer technologies have the potential to address challenges associated with performing perimetric examinations in children. For example, virtual reality–based platforms may be more comfortable for children, and they can include design features such as incorporation of game-like features and eye tracking to make the test more effective. Oculokinetic perimetry is another option for measuring visual field, especially in young children.

In contrast to adults with visual impairment, many children with visual impairment severe enough to qualify for SSA disability benefits have other comorbid health conditions. In evaluating perimetry for determining visual disability in children, it is important to allow flexibility in the requirement for formal visual field testing in children who are unable to comply with this requirement because of their developmental or health status.

Based on its review of the literature, the committee reached the following conclusion:

Conclusion 5.8: There is particular value in increased flexibility in perimetry requirements for children, given the practical considerations involved in evaluating visual field in this population across a range of ages and developmental and health statuses. Newer technologies, such as screen-based perimeters using perimetry methods that incorporate game-like features or oculokinetic perimetry, have the potential to address these challenges in pediatric perimetry and yield valid information for the identification of SSA-qualifying visual field loss.

1

Introduction

The Social Security Administration (SSA) administers the Social Security Disability Insurance (SSDI) program (under Title II of the Social Security Act) and the Supplemental Security Income (SSI) program (Title XVI of the Social Security Act). SSDI pays monthly benefits to eligible adults with disabilities who have paid into the Disability Insurance Trust Fund and are unable to work because of severe long-term disabilities, as well as to their spouses and adult children. SSI is a means-tested program based on income and financial assets that provides income assistance from U.S. Treasury general funds to adults aged 65 and older, individuals who are blind, and adults and children with disabilities.

For adults, disability is defined by statute as the "inability to do any substantial gainful activity [defined by an earnings threshold] by reason of a medically determinable physical or mental impairment [or combination of impairments] which can be expected to result in death or which has lasted or can be expected to last for a continuous period of not less than 12 months."[1] Children under age 18 are considered disabled if they have "a medically determinable physical or mental impairment, which results in marked and severe functional limitations, and which can be expected to result in death or which has lasted or can be expected to last for a continuous period of not less than 12 months."[2] A finding of disability in both adults and children depends on the severity of functional limitations arising from the claimant's impairment or combination of impairments.

---

[1] CFR § 404.1505
[2] 42 USC § 1382(c)

STUDY CHARGE AND SCOPE

In August 2024, SSA requested that the National Academies of Sciences, Engineering, and Medicine (National Academies) convene an ad hoc consensus study committee to review the latest published research and science on visual perimetry devices. The committee was charged with producing a report addressing best practices and known limitations in the use of visual perimeter devices to measure visual field loss in connection with the agency's disability evaluations. This review was to include identifying the latest standards of care regarding measurement of an individual's visual fields, as well as challenges in the provision of care. The committee also was asked to review the devices, techniques, and standards used by other federal agencies to make determinations of statutory blindness based on visual field loss. The committee's statement of task is presented in Box 1-1. Box 1-2 provides definitions for the key terms used in this report. (Additional terms appearing in the report are defined in Appendix B.)

BOX 1-1
Statement of Task

The task order objectives for the ad hoc committee of the National Academies of Sciences, Engineering, and Medicine are to review the latest published research and science and produce a report addressing best practices and known limitations in the use of visual perimeter devices to measure visual field loss in connection with disability evaluations, including

1. Describing the current practice landscape for the measurement of visual field impairment with visual perimeter devices, and recent changes or challenges in the provision of such care; and
2. Answering the following questions based on published evidence (to the extent possible) and professional judgment (where published evidence is lacking):
   a. Is optical projection of the testing stimuli still a necessity to achieve valid and reliable results from a perimeter? How does the eye respond differently to projected stimulus vs. other types (e.g., LCD screens)?
   b. Do perimeters using frequency doubling technology produce substantially similar results to traditional perimeters and what differences are there?

PREVALENCE OF VISUAL FIELD LOSS AND ITS IMPACT ON QUALITY OF LIFE

The proportion of individuals impacted by visual impairment is significant (NASEM, 2016). Based on population-level studies, approximately 4.2 million adults in the United States experience visual impairment in their better-seeing eye after correction (Varma et al., 2016). Self-reported federal survey data suggest that this number may be even higher, with nearly 8 million Americans indicating blindness or difficulty seeing even while wearing corrective lenses (Rein et al., 2022). Furthermore, an estimated 7–8 million adults have uncorrectable refractive error (Flaxman et al., 2021; Varma et al., 2016). Moreover, the prevalence of visual impairment among U.S. preschool-aged children has been estimated to be as high as 5 percent (USPSTF, 2011).

There is also evidence that the prevalence of visual impairment will increase in the future. In the United States, the number of adults who are

---

c. Is automatic kinetic perimetry a valid and reliable method of measuring visual field loss? What are the necessary device specifications and testing circumstances for automatic kinetic perimetry to produce valid and reliable visual field testing?

d. What are the most widely acceptable and commonly used alternatives to kinetic perimetry, both manual and automated, for the measurement of visual field efficiency? What impacts do such alternative methods have on the validity and reliability of testing results?

e. From a medical and practical perspective, is it still necessary for SSA to require three published clinical validation studies to find a perimeter acceptable or could fewer studies potentially show validity with similar reliability? If fewer validation studies could be acceptable, would there be higher requirements on the design or execution of those studies?

f. What devices, techniques, and standards are other federal agencies using to make statutory blindness determinations based on visual field loss?

The report will include findings and conclusions but not recommendations.

visually impaired is projected to double by 2050, affecting nearly 7 million individuals (Varma et al., 2016).

High-quality population-based studies specifically estimating the prevalence of visual field loss are rare. However, the National Health and Nutrition Examination Survey (NHANES) included visual field examination until 2008. Of 4,897 NHANES participants over the age of 40 with complete eye examinations and eye health questionnaire data, 6.83 percent displayed unilateral or bilateral visual field loss (Bernstein et al., 2024). This represents two annual cycles of NHANES data collection, each of which enrolled a nationally representative cohort.

A wider examination of NHANES data analyzed data from 3 years of surveys, including all adults 40 years of age or older without a self-reported history of refracted surgery or age-related macular degeneration (Qiu et al., 2014). Participants needed only to successfully complete a perimetry examination to be included; thus NHANES may have included disproportionately

---

BOX 1-2
Definitions of Key Terms Used in This Report

Visual field is the total area of space a person can see when the eyes are focused on a central point. It includes both central vision and peripheral vision, which is the ability to see objects to the side or up and down while looking straight ahead.

Visual field meridians refer to imaginary lines that divide the visual field into equal sections, like pieces of a pie. Typically, the visual field is divided into eight equal sections, with the meridians radiating out from the central focus point. These radii are labeled in degrees moving counterclockwise from the 3 o'clock position (0, 45, 90, 135, 180, 225, 270, and 315 degrees for an eight-meridian scheme). The radii may also be labeled using anatomical references: nasally (0 degrees in the left eye and 180 degrees in the right eye), up nasally, superiorly (90 degrees in both eyes), up temporally, temporally (180 degrees in the left eye and 0 degrees in the right eye), down temporally, inferiorly (270 degrees in both eyes), and down nasally.

Visual perimeter device (perimeter) is a machine used to measure visual fields.

Visual perimetry is the systematic measurement of visual fields.

more individuals with visual field loss. This study found that 19 percent of participants had mild, moderate, or severe visual field defects (Qiu et al., 2014).

These estimates are similar to findings in other parts of the world. For example, the Rotterdam Study evaluated 6,250 older adult residents in Rotterdam, the Netherlands, and found the overall prevalence of visual field loss to be 5.6 percent (3.0 percent in those aged 55–64 and 17.0 percent in those aged 85 or older) (Ramrattan et al., 2001). The Beijing Eye Study, which included 4,369 subjects from Beijing, China, found the visual field loss prevalence to be 5.3 percent in subjects aged 40–49 and 25.4 percent in those aged 70 and older (Wang et al., 2006).

Visual field loss is associated with a number of conditions, including glaucoma, macular degeneration, retinal vascular occlusive disease, stroke, optic nerve conditions such as optic neuritis, and inherited retinal diseases such as retinitis pigmentosa. Visual field loss has a significant impact on quality of life and can result in varying degrees of disability, particularly with

---

Automated perimetry refers to automated presentation of the test stimulus and recording of patient responses.

Static perimetry refers to stationary stimuli presented at defined points in the visual field. Locations at which the stimulus is seen and not seen are recorded.

Threshold refers to the stimulus intensity that a person can detect on 50 percent of presentations.

Kinetic perimetry uses a moving stimulus that is generally moved from a nonseeing area to a seeing area in a systematic way to map the central and peripheral visual field boundaries, in addition to any scotomas, including blind spots. This movement can be automated, semiautomated, or manual.

Static automated threshold perimetry (static or standard automated perimetry),[a] or "white-on-white perimetry," refers to the projection of a stationary white stimulus onto a white background to determine the probable threshold at chosen locations in the visual field. Blue on yellow static automated threshold perimetry is also available.

Automated (or automatic) kinetic perimetry[b] uses a moving stimulus of a selected size and intensity, with the speed and direction of the stimulus being automated.

continued

> **BOX 1-2 Continued**
>
> **Optical projection** consists of projecting a light stimulus onto a background to present it to the patient's eye in order to map the visual field.
>
> **Frequency doubling technology,** used in some perimeters, is based on a flicker illusion, which essentially creates an image that appears double its actual spatial frequency. The stimulus does not move across the field, and the flickering is a proxy for the stimulus intensity used in either static or kinetic perimetry.
>
> **Visual acuity** is a measure of the sharpness or clarity of vision at a given distance.
>
> **Visual acuity efficiency** (Social Security Administration [SSA] definition) is expressed as a percentage corresponding to the best-corrected central visual acuity for distance in the better eye, based on a reference chart that aligns Snellen visual acuity metrics with visual acuity efficiency percentages (SSA, n.d.-a, 2.00A7b).
>
> **Visual acuity impairment value** (SSA definition) is a value corresponding to the best-corrected central visual acuity for distance in the better eye, based on a reference chart using Snellen metrics.
>
> **Visual field efficiency** (SSA definition) is expressed as a percentage corresponding to the visual field in the better eye, calculated by adding the number of degrees seen along the eight principal meridians found on a visual field chart and dividing by 5. For example, if the visual field is contracted down to 25 degrees in all eight meridians, the remaining visual field efficiency would be $25 \times 8 \div 5 = 40$ percent (SSA, n.d.-a, 2.00A7c).
>
> **Visual field impairment value** (SSA definition) is a value corresponding to the visual field in a person's better eye. It is calculated by dividing the

respect to daily functioning, including the ability to work; social engagement; and emotional well-being. Survey measures have been developed to quantitatively assess health-related quality of life (HRQoL) both in general and in the context of a person's visual health. Cross-sectional and prospective studies found that both types of HRQoL measures varied linearly with visual field extent (McKean-Cowdin et al., 2007; Patino et al., 2011).

There have also been studies characterizing the impact of visual field loss on specific aspects of individuals' lives. Individuals with moderate to absolute value of the mean deviation from acceptable static automated threshold perimetry by 22 (SSA, n.d.-a).

Mean deviation is the average difference in visual field sensitivity across all measured locations compared with a normal, age-matched reference field.

Visual efficiency (SSA definition) is a calculated value of a person's remaining visual function. Expressed as a percentage, it is calculated by multiplying an individual's visual acuity efficiency percentage by their visual field efficiency percentage and dividing by 100. For example, if the visual acuity efficiency percentage is 75 and the visual field efficiency percentage is 40, the visual efficiency percentage is (75 × 40) / 100 = 30 percent (SSA, n.d.-a).

Visual impairment value (SSA definition) is a calculated value of a person's loss of visual function, which is calculated by adding their visual acuity impairment value and their visual field impairment value (SSA, n.d.-a).

Statutory blindness refers to blindness as defined in the Social Security Act: (1) "central visual acuity of 20/200 or less in the better eye with the use of a correcting lens" or (2) "an eye that has a visual field limitation such that the widest diameter of the visual field subtends an angle no greater than 20 degrees" (Social Security Act, sections 216[i][1]; 1614[a][2]).

SOURCES: CHOP (n.d.); EyeWiki (2023, 2024); Medline Plus (2023); SSA (n.d.-a, -c).

---

[a] Multiple terms are used to refer to the same technology. This report preferentially uses the term *static automated threshold perimetry* to distinguish it from other types of perimetry (e.g., kinetic, manual, suprathreshold).

[b] Although *automated (or automatic) kinetic perimetry* is typically used in the literature, this report preferentially uses the term *semiautomated kinetic perimetry* to be more precise about the role of the technician in administering the test (see Chapter 5).

---

severe visual field loss may have difficulty performing routine tasks such as moving about and navigating different environments, as well as driving and reading, which leads in turn to greater reliance on others and reduced independence (Qiu et al., 2014; Turano et al., 2004). The loss can heighten the risk of injury due to impaired peripheral vision, making bumping into objects and falls more common (Patino et al., 2010; Qiu et al., 2014; Turano et al., 2004). Furthermore, studies show that people with visual field loss often suffer from a decline in mental health, including symptoms of anxiety and depression, as they adapt to their diminished vision (Wang et al., 2017). Visual field loss also limits the ability to engage in social activities, thereby reducing overall social participation and contributing to feelings of isolation (Lange et al., 2021). The degree of impact varies depending on the severity of the field loss, with more profound impairment leading to greater disability and poorer quality of life (Qiu et al., 2014). Furthermore, when coupled with other chronic conditions that affect many working adults (e.g., depression, stroke, cardiac conditions), visual field loss significantly increases the potential impact of these conditions on a person's ability to perform various tasks (NASEM, 2016).

SSA'S DISABILILTY EVALUATION PROCESS[3]

SSA uses a five-step process based on medical–vocational evaluations to determine whether an adult meets the definition of disability. After SSA determines an applicant's administrative eligibility and the presence of a medical impairment of sufficient duration and severity in steps 1 and 2 of this process, it assesses, in step 3, whether the applicant's impairment meets or medically equals the criteria listed for a condition in SSA's (n.d.-b) Listing of Impairments-Adult Listings (listings). The Adult Listings are organized by major body system and describe impairments that SSA considers to be sufficiently severe to prevent an applicant from performing any gainful activity, regardless of age, education, or work experience. Step 3 is used as a "screen-in" step, meaning if an individual is not found to qualify for disability benefits at this step, they are not denied; rather, the assessment moves on to step 4. If an impairment is severe but does not meet or medically equal any listing, SSA assesses in step 4 whether the applicant's physical or mental residual functional capacity allows the person to perform past relevant work. Applicants who are able to perform past relevant work are denied benefits, while those who are unable to do so proceed to step 5. At step 5, SSA considers, in combination with the applicant's residual functional capacity, such vocational factors as age, education, and work experience, including transferable skills, in determining whether the individual can perform other work in the national economy. Applicants determined to be unable to adjust to performing other work are allowed benefits, while those determined able to adjust are denied.

Disability determinations in children follow a three-step sequential evaluation process. After determining administrative eligibility and the presence of a medical impairment of sufficient duration and severity, SSA assesses in step 3 whether the impairment(s) meets, medically equals (is equivalent

---

[3] The text in this section is taken from NASEM, 2022, pp. 14–15.

in severity to), or functionally equals (i.e., the impairment[s] results in functional limitations equivalent in severity to) the criteria in SSA's (n.d.-d) Child Listings.[4] If a child's impairment or combination of impairments "does not meet or medically equal any listing, [SSA] will decide whether it results in limitations that functionally equal the listings."[5] SSA refers to limitations that functionally equal the listings as being functionally equivalent to the listings. SSA's technique for determining functional equivalence is a "whole child" approach that "accounts for all of the effects of a child's impairments singly and in combination—the interactive and cumulative effects of the impairments—because it starts with a consideration of actual functioning in all settings" (SSA, 2009, p. 7527).

For both adults and children, disability claims related to visual field loss are evaluated under listings for the Special Senses and Speech body system.[6]

SSA'S CURRENT STANDARDS FOR MEASURING VISUAL FIELDS

The Special Senses and Speech listings for both adults and children (SSA, n.d.-a, 2.00; n.d.-c, 102.00) specify criteria for the evaluation of visual disorders for the purposes of SSA disability determinations. These criteria describe the degree of impairment necessary for an individual to qualify for disability benefits because of their eyesight alone. These criteria, and the associated introductory text in the listing, include requirements for how visual field loss must be measured in order to meet the criteria. Generally, SSA requires that visual field testing, or perimetry, be carried out using automated static threshold perimetry[7] performed on a perimeter meeting defined requirements. Kinetic perimetry meeting similarly defined requirements can also be used unless a specific listing states otherwise, or an applicant's impairment results in a significant limitation in the central visual field. SSA also has a specific criterion using a metric called visual field efficiency, which can only be measured with kinetic perimetry.

Within the Special Senses and Speech listings, there are six pathways through which individuals can qualify for disability benefits because of visual impairment (see Table 1-1). Each pathway refers to a benchmark for visual acuity, visual field diameter, or both. Annex Table 1-1 contains

---

[4] 20 CFR § 416.926; 20 CFR § 416.926a
[5] 20 CFR § 416.926a
[6] The Special Senses and Speech listings for adults are available at https://www.ssa.gov/disability/professionals/bluebook/2.00-SpecialSensesandSpeech-Adult.htm (accessed January 28, 2025). Those for children are available at https://www.ssa.gov/disability/professionals/bluebook/102.00-SpecialSensesandSpeech-Childhood.htm (accessed January 28, 2025).
[7] Automated static threshold perimetry is the same as static automated threshold perimetry, which is the term this report uses preferentially.

TABLE 1-1 Summary of Pathways to Meeting the Social Security Administration's Listing Criteria for Visual Disorders

SSA Listing Section	Description	Static vs. Kinetic Perimetry	Testing Requirement	Meets Criteria for Statutory Blindness	Qualifies for SSA Disability Benefits
2.02	Central visual acuity of 20/200 or less in the better eye with correction	n/a	Testing with Snellen eye chart or comparable testing methodology	Yes	Yes
2.03A	Widest visual field diameter (through central fixation) no greater than 20 degrees	Static automated threshold perimetry; manual or semiautomated kinetic perimetry	Size III/4e stimulus and white background (31.5 asb)	Yes	Yes
2.03B	Mean deviation of 22 decibels or greater in the central 30 degrees of the visual field (30 degrees from the point of fixation)	Static automated threshold perimetry	Automated static threshold perimetry with a white size III stimulus, using 30-2 pattern	No	Yes
2.03C	Visual field efficiency of 20 percent or less	Manual or semiautomated kinetic perimetry	Size III/4e stimulus across 8 principal meridians	No	Yes
2.04A	Visual efficiency (VAE × VFE ÷ 100) of 20 percent or less after best correction	See Section 2.03C	See Sections 2.02 and 2.03C	No	Yes
2.04B	Visual impairment (VAI + VFI) of 1.0 or greater	See Section 2.03B	See Sections 2.02 and 2.03B	No	Yes

NOTES: asb = apostilb; VAE = visual acuity efficiency; VAI = visual acuity impairment value; VFE = visual field efficiency; VFI = visual field impairment value.
SOURCES: SSA (n.d.-a, -c).

selected excerpts relevant to visual field testing from the listings and another SSA policy document.

Two of the six pathways refer to the federal definition of statutory blindness. Meeting the criteria for statutory blindness requires either "central visual acuity of 20/200 or less in the better eye with the use of a correcting lens" (SSA, n.d.-a, 2.00A2a; n.d.-c, 102.02) or "a visual field limitation such that the widest diameter of the visual field [does not exceed]

20 degrees" (SSA, n.d.-a, 2.03A; n.d.-c, 102.03A). Individuals who satisfy the criteria for statutory blindness automatically qualify for SSA disability benefits. Qualification for benefits under the visual field definition of statutory blindness in Section 2.03A requires the use of a visual field test measuring the central 24–30 degrees from the point of fixation. No specific method is mentioned beyond that requirement, meaning that any static or kinetic perimetric method otherwise accepted by SSA can be used to qualify for disability benefits under Section 2.03A.

Individuals who do not meet the criteria for statutory blindness may still qualify for disability benefits under alternative provisions, including Sections 2.03B, 2.03C, 2.04A, or 2.04B. These provisions account for cases in which visual acuity and visual field loss fall short of the stricter statutory blindness definition but still demonstrate significant impairment. Sections 2.03B and 2.03C consider visual field extent alone, while Sections 2.04A and 2.04B consider visual field extent and visual acuity combined. Importantly, SSA policies note that qualifying for disability benefits under one of these sections does *not* mean an applicant is legally blind, a designation that holds a specific meaning throughout the statute.

Section 2.03B refers to a metric called mean deviation or mean defect. Mean deviation, typically reported in decibels (dB), reflects the average loss of sensitivity across a person's visual field, using the typical visual field as a standard. In perimetry, stimulus intensity is measured in dB. At different locations in the visual field, a person may not be able to see stimuli of lesser intensity. The deviation at a single location in the visual field is the difference between the minimum intensity the *examinee* can see and the minimum intensity a *typical person* can see.

Mean deviation is the average deviation in sensitivity across all measured visual field locations. For a determination of disability under Section 2.03B, SSA requires measurements from automated static threshold perimetry (SSA, n.d.-a, 2.00A6d). Section 2.03B requires "automated static threshold perimetry," also known as static automated perimetry, which displays a stimulus at different locations in the examinee's field of view. The examinee indicates when they see the stimulus, and the perimeter statistically calculates the extent of the examinee's visual field. Chapter 3 provides a more detailed discussion of the methodology of static automated threshold perimetry. For the purposes of Section 2.03B, the perimeter used must also measure the central 30 degrees of the visual field. If, within those central 30 degrees, an applicant's mean deviation is 22 dB or worse, they will qualify for disability benefits under this section.

For determination of disability under Section 2.03C, SSA considers a measurement known as visual field efficiency (SSA, n.d.-a, 2.00A7c). Visual field efficiency essentially corresponds to the percentage of a typical visual field that a person can see through their better eye. SSA calculates visual field efficiency by summing the number of degrees at which the examinee can see a stimulus across each of eight "principal meridians" of the eye and then dividing by 5. The principal meridians are located at 0, 45, 90, 135, 180, 225, 270, and 315 degrees radially around the eye, moving counterclockwise from 3 o'clock (Figure 1-1). Since the typical visual field will have a sum of 500 degrees across its principal meridians, dividing the sum by 5 yields a percentage for visual field efficiency. A visual field efficiency of 20 percent or less qualifies an applicant for disability benefits under Section 2.03C. As noted above, measurement of visual field efficiency requires the use of kinetic perimetry, the methodology for which is discussed in Chapter 5.

Sections 2.04A and 2.04B allow for a determination of disability based on combined metrics of visual acuity and visual field loss. These pathways ensure that individuals with extensive visual field loss or combined impairments can still be assessed fairly. Parallel listings for children can be found in Sections 102.03 and 102.04.

Section 2.04A references a measure called visual efficiency, not to be confused with visual field efficiency (SSA, n.d.-a, 2.00A7d). Visual efficiency is a broader measure that includes both visual field efficiency and visual acuity efficiency. Visual acuity efficiency is determined using a reference

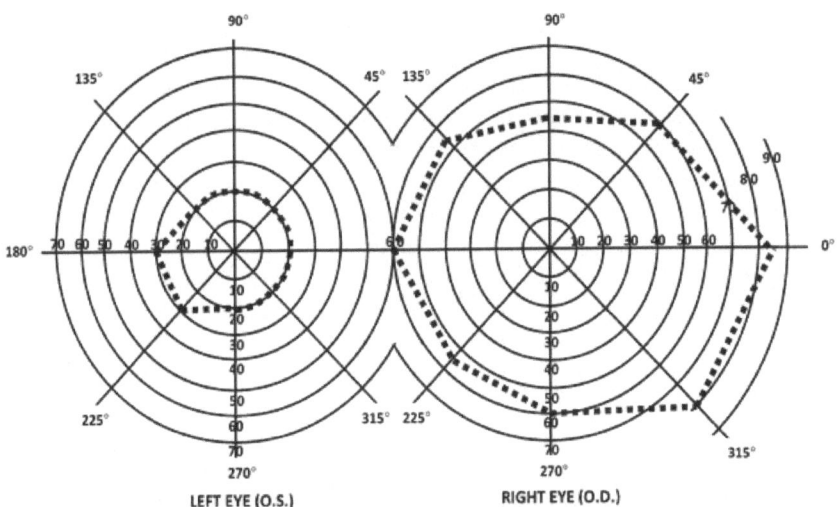

FIGURE 1-1 Diagram of the eight principal meridians for each eye.
NOTE: The diagram for the right eye shows a typical visual field extent drawn in dashed lines. The diagram for the left eye shows a constrained visual field; a healthy visual field would be a mirror image of the right eye's field shape. In addition, the degrees assigned to each meridian are *not* mirrored and instead remain the same.
SOURCE: SSA (n.d.-a, 2.00A7cB).

chart that aligns Snellen visual acuity metrics with visual acuity efficiency percentages (e.g., 20/20 corresponds to 100 percent; 20/100 corresponds to 50 percent) (SSA, n.d.-a, 2.00A7b). Visual efficiency is calculated by multiplying an applicant's visual field efficiency by their visual acuity efficiency and dividing by 100. A visual efficiency of less than 20 percent after best correction qualifies a person for disability benefits under Section 2.04A. Since the calculation of visual efficiency requires a measure of visual field efficiency, it, too, requires the use of kinetic perimetry.

Finally, Section 2.04B references a measure called visual impairment value. The visual impairment value is the sum of the "impairment values" for both visual acuity and visual field (see SSA, n.d.-a, 2.00A8d). The visual field impairment value is the mean deviation, calculated using static automated threshold perimetry as for Section 2.03B, divided by 22. The visual acuity impairment value is read from a reference chart using Snellen metrics (SSA, n.d.-a, 2.00A8b). If the sum of these two impairment values is 1.00 after best correction or greater, the applicant qualifies for disability benefits.

STUDY APPROACH

To carry out its charge, the committee met four times to discuss the questions posed in the statement of task (Box 1-1). At the second meeting, a public information-gathering session was held, in which speakers were invited for three panel discussions. The discussion topics were disparities and opportunities in access to vision testing, lived experiences with visual impairment and applying for SSA disability benefits, and emerging technologies in visual field testing.

The panel on disparities and opportunities in access to vision testing, along with the lived experiences panel, guided the committee's understanding of challenges in providing care. Through these panels, the committee heard how visual impairment can affect employment, day-to-day life, and general well-being. Specifically, the committee heard about the vastly different experiences of panelists who needed visual field tests to qualify for SSA disability benefits with respect to whether they were able to receive such tests or whether such a test was even offered. As a result, some panelists experienced increased confusion while navigating their condition and the SSDI application process, and in some cases, panelists' diagnosis or approval for benefits was delayed. Panelists also discussed how cost, unfamiliarity with screening devices, and the possible need to visit more than one clinician for treatment were barriers to receiving vision care.

Focusing on the specific difficulties people encounter when applying for disability due to vision impairment became a helpful framing for the committee. SSA requires that applicants' medical records include certain documentation and test results related to their disabilities. If the required tests are not accessible, an individual may find it difficult or even impossible to be approved for disability benefits.

Some perimetry devices are less expensive than others for clinics to acquire or use, or they may not have personnel properly trained to use some perimeters. Other devices are easier for the examinee to use comfortably. In some cases, the only clinic accessible to an applicant has only a perimeter deemed unacceptable by SSA. A central goal of the committee in developing this report was to aid SSA in understanding how best to broaden the scope of acceptable perimeters while maintaining standards of reliability and validity. The committee was also guided by a previous National Academies report, *Visual Impairments: Determining Eligibility for Social Security Benefits* (NRC, 2002).

For each of the specific questions in the statement of task, National Academies staff aided committee members in conducting literature searches. The committee then discussed and reached consensus on conclusions for each question based on the published evidence, and where such evidence was lacking, the committee members' professional judgment. Additionally, staff performed a broad scoping search of perimetry validation studies published since 2002. This review supported the committee's discussion of essential elements of an effective perimetry validation study while helping to ensure that those standards were achievable. The key words used in the search were ("visual field test*" OR perimetry) AND validat*. Included were studies assessing or validating new perimeters and comparison of perimeters. Excluded were studies not analyzing perimetry, those using perimetry but that do not have a standard reference comparator, structure–function papers, analysis of data or statistical modeling of existing perimeters, deep learning models, and vision-related activity scales. Searches in Medline, Scopus, and Embase yielded 832 results after duplicates were eliminated. Committee members and staff screened those papers, narrowing those results down to 68 papers for review.

ORGANIZATION OF THE REPORT

Chapter 2 addresses the topic of which devices, techniques, and standards other federal agencies are using to make statutory blindness determinations based on visual field loss. Chapter 3 introduces basic concepts in perimetry and provides an overview of current practice in the measurement of visual fields, recent changes in practice, variability and challenges in the measurement of visual fields, and new technologies that could ameliorate some of the systems-level challenges. Chapter 4 reviews key considerations in evaluating new perimetry techniques. Chapter 5 responds to some of the specific topics in the statement of task, including optical projection, static compared with kinetic perimetry, alternatives to kinetic perimetry for measuring visual field efficiency, frequency doubling technology, and specific considerations for pediatric populations.

REFERENCES

Bernstein, I. A., A. C. Fisher, K. Singh, and S. Y. Wang. 2024. The association between frailty and visual field loss in US adults. *American Journal of Ophthalmology* 257 (January):38–45.

CHOP (Children's Hospital of Philadelphia). n.d. *Functional vision*. https://www.chop.edu/conditions-diseases/functional-vision (accessed January 29, 2025).

EyeWiki. 2023. *Frequency doubling technology*. https://eyewiki.org/Frequency_Doubling_Technology (accessed January 29, 2025).

EyeWiki. 2024. *Standard automated perimetry*. https://eyewiki.org/Standard_Automated_Perimetry#Manual_vs._Automated_Perimetry (accessed January 29, 2025).

Flaxman, A. D., J. S. Wittenborn, T. Robalik, R. Gulia, R. B. Gerzoff, E. A. Lundeen, J. Saaddine, D. B. Rein, and Vision and Eye Health Surveillance System Study Group. 2021. Prevalence of visual acuity loss or blindness in the US: A Bayesian meta-analysis. *JAMA Ophthalmology* 139(7):717–723.

Lange, R., A. Kumagai, S. Weiss, K. B. Zaffke, S. Day, D. Wicker, A. Howson, K. T. Jayasundera, L. Smolinski, and C. Hedlich. 2021. Vision-related quality of life in adults with severe peripheral vision loss: A qualitative interview study. *Journal of Patient-Reported Outcomes* 5:1–12.

McKean-Cowdin, R., R. Varma, J. Wu, R. D. Hays, and S. P. Azen. 2007. Severity of visual field loss and health-related quality of life. *American Journal of Ophthalmology* 143(6):1013–1023.

Medline Plus. 2023. *Visual field*. https://medlineplus.gov/ency/article/003879.htm (accessed January 29, 2025).

NASEM (National Academies of Sciences, Engineering, and Medicine). 2016. *Making eye health a population health imperative: Vision for tomorrow*. Washington, DC: The National Academies Press.

NASEM. 2022. *Selected heritable disorders of connective tissues and disability*. Washington, DC: The National Academies Press.

NRC (National Research Council). 2002. *Visual impairments: Determining eligibility for Social Security benefits*. Washington, DC: The National Academy Press.

Patino, C. M., R. McKean-Cowdin, S. P. Azen, J. C. Allison, F. Choudhury, R. Varma, and Los Angeles Latino Eye Study Group. 2010. Central and peripheral visual impairment and the risk of falls and falls with injury. *Ophthalmology* 117(2):199–206.e1.

Patino, C. M., R. Varma, S. P. Azen, D. V. Conti, M. B. Nichol, and R. McKean-Cowdin. 2011. The impact of change in visual field on health-related quality of life the Los Angeles Latino eye study. *Ophthalmology* 118(7):1310–1317.

Qiu, M., S. Y. Wang, K. Singh, and S. C. Lin. 2014. Association between visual field defects and quality of life in the United States. *Ophthalmology* 121(3):733–740.

Ramrattan, R. S., R. C. Wolfs, S. Panda-Jonas, J. B. Jonas, D. Bakker, H. A. Pols, A. Hofman, and P. T. de Jong. 2001. Prevalence and causes of visual field loss in the elderly and associations with impairment in daily functioning: The Rotterdam study. *Archives of Ophthalmology* 119(12):1788–1794.

Rein, D. B., J. S. Wittenborn, P. Zhang, F. Sublett, P. A. Lamuda, E. A. Lundeen, and J. Saaddine. 2022. The economic burden of vision loss and blindness in the United States. *Ophthalmology* 129(4):369–378.

SSA (U.S. Social Security Administration). 2007. SRR 07-01p: Titles II and XVI: Evaluating visual field loss using automated static threshold perimetry. *Federal Register* 72(146):41796. https://www.ssa.gov/OP_Home/rulings/di/01/SSR2007-01-di-01.html (accessed February 3, 2025).

SSA. 2009. SSR 09-1p: Title XVI: Determining childhood disability under the functional equivalence rule—The "whole child" approach. *Federal Register* 74(30):7527. https://www.ssa.gov/OP_Home/rulings/ssi/02/SSR2009-01-ssi-02.html (accessed January 28, 2025).

SSA. n.d.-a. *Disability evaluation under Social Security—2.00 special senses and speech—Adult.* https://www.ssa.gov/disability/professionals/bluebook/2.00-SpecialSensesandSpeech-Adult.htm (accessed February 3, 2025).

SSA. n.d.-b. *Disability evaluation under Social Security—Listing of impairments—Adult listings (Part A).* https://www.ssa.gov/disability/professionals/bluebook/AdultListings.htm (accessed January 28, 2025).

SSA. n.d.-c. *Disability evaluation under Social Security—102.00 special senses and speech—Childhood.* https://www.ssa.gov/disability/professionals/bluebook/102.00-SpecialSensesandSpeech-Childhood.htm (accessed February 3, 2025).

SSA. n.d.-d. *Disability evaluation under Social Security—Listing of impairments—Childhood listings (Part B).* https://www.ssa.gov/disability/professionals/bluebook/ChildhoodListings.htm (accessed January 28, 2025).

Turano, K. A., A. T. Broman, K. Bandeen-Roche, B. Munoz, G. S. Rubin, S. West, and SEE Project Team. 2004. Association of visual field loss and mobility performance in older adults: Salisbury Eye Evaluation Study. *Optometry and Vision Science* 81(5):298–307.

USPSTF (U.S. Preventive Services Task Force). 2011. *Evidence summary: Visual impairment in children ages 1-5: Screening.* https://www.uspreventiveservicestaskforce.org/uspstf/document/evidence-summary5/visual-impairment-in-children-ages-1-5-screening-2011

Varma, R., T. S. Vajaranant, B. Burkemper, S. Wu, M. Torres, C. Hsu, F. Choudhury, and R. McKean-Cowdin. 2016. Visual impairment and blindness in adults in the United States: Demographic and geographic variations from 2015 to 2050. *JAMA Ophthalmology* 134(7):802–809.

Wang, Y., L. Xu, and J. B. Jonas. 2006. Prevalence and causes of visual field loss as determined by frequency doubling perimetry in urban and rural adult Chinese. *American Journal of Ophthalmology* 141(6):1078–1086.

Wang, Y., S. Alnwisi, and M. Ke. 2017. The impact of mild, moderate, and severe visual field loss in glaucoma on patients' quality of life measured via the Glaucoma Quality of Life-15 questionnaire: A meta-analysis. *Medicine* 96(48):e8019.

INTRODUCTION

ANNEX TABLE 1-1 Selected Excerpts Relevant to Visual Field Testing from Social Security Administration Documents

Reference	Excerpted text
2.00 (Adult)[a] 102.00 (Child)	
2.00A6a 102.00A6a	6. *How do we measure visual fields?* a. *General.* We generally need visual field testing when you have a visual disorder that could result in visual field loss, such as glaucoma, retinitis pigmentosa, or optic neuropathy, or when you display behaviors that suggest a visual field loss. When we need to measure the extent of your visual field loss, we use visual field testing (also referred to as perimetry) carried out using automated static threshold perimetry performed on an acceptable perimeter.
2.00A6c 102.00A6c	c. *Evaluation under* 2.03A. To determine statutory blindness based on visual field loss in your better eye (2.03A), we need the results of a visual field test that measures the central 24 to 30 degrees of your visual field; that is, the area measuring 24 to 30 degrees from the point of fixation. Acceptable tests include the Humphrey Field Analyzer (HFA) 30-2, HFA 24-2, and Octopus 32.
2.00A6d 102.00A6d	d. *Evaluation under* 2.03B. To determine whether your visual field loss meets listing 2.03B, we use the mean deviation or defect (MD) from acceptable automated static threshold perimetry that measures the central 30 degrees of the visual field. MD is the average sensitivity deviation from normal values for all measured visual field locations. When using results from HFA tests, which report the MD as a negative number, we use the absolute value of the MD to determine whether your visual field loss meets listing 2.03B. We cannot use tests that do not measure the central 30 degrees of the visual field, such as the HFA 24-2, to determine if your impairment meets or medically equals 2.03B.
2.00A9 102.00A9	9. *What are our requirements for an acceptable perimeter?* We will use results from automated static threshold perimetry performed on a perimeter that: a. Uses optical projection to generate the test stimuli. b. Has an internal normative database for automatically comparing your performance with that of the general population. c. Has a statistical analysis package that is able to calculate visual field indices, particularly MD. d. Demonstrates the ability to correctly detect visual field loss and correctly identify normal visual fields. e. Demonstrates good test-retest reliability. f. Has undergone clinical validation studies by three or more independent laboratories with results published in peer-reviewed ophthalmic journals.

continued

ANNEX TABLE 1-1 Continued

Reference	Excerpted text
2.00A6b 02.00A6b	b. *Automated static threshold perimetry requirements.* (i) The test must use a white size III Goldmann stimulus and a 31.5 apostilb (asb) white background (or a 10 candela per square meter (cd/m^2) white background). The stimuli test locations must be no more than 6 degrees apart horizontally or vertically. Measurements must be reported on standard charts and include a description of the size and intensity of the test stimulus. (ii) We measure the extent of your visual field loss by determining the portion of the visual field in which you can see a white III4e stimulus. The "III" refers to the standard Goldmann test stimulus size III (4 mm^2), and the "4e" refers to the standard Goldmann intensity filter (0 decibel (dB) attenuation, which allows presentation of the maximum luminance) used to determine the intensity of the stimulus. (iii) In automated static threshold perimetry, the intensity of the stimulus varies. The intensity of the stimulus is expressed in decibels (dB). A perimeter's maximum stimulus luminance is usually assigned the value 0 dB. We need to determine the dB level that corresponds to a 4e intensity for the particular perimeter being used. We will then use the dB printout to determine which points you see at a 4e intensity level (a "seeing point"). [Examples are provided in the full listing referenced here.]
2.00A7 102.00A7	7. *How do we determine your visual acuity efficiency, visual field efficiency, and visual efficiency?* a. *General. Visual efficiency*, a calculated value of your remaining visual function, is the combination of your *visual acuity efficiency* and your *visual field efficiency* expressed as a percentage. b. *Visual acuity efficiency.* Visual acuity efficiency is a percentage that corresponds to the best-corrected central visual acuity for distance in your better eye. See Table 1. [Table 1 is included in the full listing referenced here.] c. *Visual field efficiency.* Visual field efficiency is a percentage that corresponds to the visual field in your better eye. Under 2.03C, we require kinetic perimetry to determine your visual field efficiency percentage. We calculate the visual field efficiency percentage by adding the number of degrees you see along the eight principal meridians found on a visual field chart (0, 45, 90, 135, 180, 225, 270, and 315) in your better eye and dividing by 5. [Examples are provided in the full listing referenced here.] d. *Visual efficiency.* Under 2.04A, we calculate the visual efficiency percentage by multiplying your visual acuity efficiency percentage (see 2.00A7b) by your visual field efficiency percentage (see 2.00A7c) and dividing by 100. For example, if your visual acuity efficiency percentage is 75 and your visual field efficiency percentage is 36, your visual efficiency percentage is: (75 × 36) / 100 = 27 percent.

ANNEX TABLE 1-1 Continued

Reference	Excerpted text
2.00A6e 102.00A6e	e. *Other types of perimetry.* If the evidence in your case contains visual field measurements obtained using manual or automated kinetic perimetry, such as Goldmann perimetry or the HFA "SSA Test Kinetic," we can generally use these results if the kinetic test was performed using a white III4e stimulus projected on a white 31.5 asb (10 cd/m^2) background. Automated kinetic perimetry, such as the HFA "SSA Test Kinetic," does not detect limitations in the central visual field because testing along a meridian stops when you see the stimulus. If your visual disorder has progressed to the point at which it is likely to result in a significant limitation in the central visual field, such as a scotoma (see 2.00A6h), we will not use *automated* kinetic perimetry to determine the extent of your visual field loss. Instead, we will determine the extent of your visual field loss using automated static threshold perimetry or manual kinetic perimetry.
2.00A6g 102.00A6g	g. *Use of corrective lenses.* You must not wear eyeglasses during visual field testing because they limit your field of vision. You may wear contact lenses to correct your visual acuity during the visual field test to obtain the most accurate visual field measurements. For this single purpose, you do not need to demonstrate that you have the ability to use the contact lenses on a sustained basis.
2.00A6h 102.00A6h	h. *Scotoma.* A scotoma is a field defect or non-seeing area (also referred to as a "blind spot") in the visual field surrounded by a normal field or seeing area. When we measure your visual field, we subtract the length of any scotoma, other than the normal blind spot, from the overall length of any diameter on which it falls.
2.02 102.02	*Loss of Central Visual Acuity.* Remaining vision in the better eye after best correction is 20/200 or less.
2.03 102.03	*Contraction of the visual field in the better eye,* with: A. The widest diameter subtending an angle around the point of fixation no greater than 20 degrees; OR B. An MD of 22 decibels or greater, determined by automated static threshold perimetry that measures the central 30 degrees of the visual field (see 2.00A6d). OR C. A visual field efficiency of 20 percent or less, determined by kinetic perimetry (see 2.00A7c).
2.04 102.04	*Loss of visual efficiency, or visual impairment, in the better eye:* A. A visual efficiency percentage of 20 or less after best correction (see 2.00A7d). OR B. A visual impairment value of 1.00 or greater after best correction (see 2.00A8d).

continued

ANNEX TABLE 1-1 Continued

Reference	Excerpted text
SSR 07-01p	
Policy Interpretation, Step 2	*Step 2—Are the test results reliable?*
	Each perimeter manufacturer will identify factors that are used to determine whether the test results are reliable.
	For the Humphrey Field Analyzer, the reliability factors are fixation losses, false positive errors, and false negative errors. Information about these factors is at the top of the chart (see Exhibits 1 and 2). The test results are not reliable for evaluating visual field loss if the fixation losses exceed 20 percent, or if the false positive errors or false negative errors exceed 33 percent.
	Even when the reliability factors are within the manufacturer's specifications, we will not use the test results to evaluate visual field loss if there is other information in the case file that suggests that the results are not valid; for example, the test results are inconsistent with the clinical findings or the individual's daily activities.

[a]The original source contains links to other portions of the 2.00 Special Senses and Speech—Adult listing.
SOURCES: SSA (n.d.-a,-c; 2007).

2

How Other Selected Federal Agencies Assess Impairment Due to Visual Field Loss

Like the Social Security Administration (SSA), many government agencies have their own definitions of visual impairment and acceptable methods for assessing visual field loss. Assessments using these standards determine eligibility for disability benefits, eligibility for other disability-related programs, or qualification for jobs. Both definitions of visual impairment and assessment methods deemed acceptable vary between agencies.

Most agency definitions go beyond the federal definition of statutory blindness due to field loss, which requires that the widest diameter of a person's visual field be 20 degrees or less at the visual horizon—in other words, 10 degrees in either direction from the point of central fixation. Some agencies, similarly to SSA, use statutory blindness as one of several criteria a person can meet to qualify as having a disability. Others adopt a functional definition of visual disability based on potential obstacles to engaging in relevant daily tasks. Most, however, set a specific visual field size that examinees must meet or not meet. The preferred perimeters and measurement techniques vary as well, with some permitting a broader selection of devices and techniques than others. Some of these differences are task specific and may involve stricter guidelines when safety is a concern. Stringent requirements can be found outside of occupational testing, such as in state-by-state visual requirements for driver's licensure. However, the committee found many of these differences to be arbitrary.

The sections below review the criteria and methods used by selected federal agencies other than SSA for purposes of determining qualification for disability benefits, determining eligibility for employment in jobs that require good vision, and measuring functional vision.

DISABILITY BENEFITS

Like SSA, certain other federal and state agencies assess visual field loss to determine whether a person has a compensable disability. These agencies typically have the most rigorous and well-defined requirements for visual field measurement.

Department of Veterans Affairs

The Department of Veterans Affairs assesses the nature and severity of veterans' service-related disabilities. These assessments result in "disability ratings," expressed in percentages, that affect the monthly amount of a veteran's disability compensation, as well as their eligibility for other benefits and programs.

The perimeter requirements[1] of the Department of Veterans Affairs are very similar to those used by SSA for disability determination. For disability rating, visual field evaluation requires the use of manual or semi-automated kinetic perimeters, specifically "Goldmann [manual] kinetic perimetry or [semi]automated [kinetic] perimetry using Humphrey Model 750, Octopus Model 101, or later versions of these perimetric devices with simulated kinetic Goldmann testing capability."[2] These perimeters also meet SSA's requirements for semiautomated kinetic perimetry. Also like SSA, the Department of Veterans Affairs requires that perimeters use the Goldmann III/4e stimulus. However, certain aphakic (lacking a lens) or pseudophakic (having an artificial lens implanted) veterans are allowed to use a IV/4e stimulus, which is larger. The Department of Veterans Affairs averages an individual's remaining visual field (measured in degrees) across the eight principal meridians of the eye to determine the average concentric contraction of the visual field in each eye. Lower average concentric contractions result in higher disability ratings.

Office of Workers' Compensation Programs

The Department of Labor's Office of Workers' Compensation Programs (OWCP) administers four federal workers' compensation programs, each covering a different group of employees. Two of these—the Federal Employees' Compensation Program and the Longshore Program—compensate employees who permanently lose limbs, organs, or their functions. For both of these programs, the loss of 80 percent or more of visual function is considered the same as completely losing the eye.[3]

---

[1] CFR § 4.77
[2] CFR § 4.77
[3] See 5 USC § 8107(c) and 33 USC § 908(c).

The percentage loss of visual function is calculated using the American Medical Association's (AMA's) *Guides to the Evaluation of Permanent Impairment* (AMA, 2024). The sixth edition of the *Guides* assigns a visual field score based on the number of points along each of 10 meridians that a person can see. These meridians are different from the "eight principal meridians" referenced in SSA's listings. The meridians in the *Guides* are located at 25, 65, 115, 155, 195, 225, 255, 285, 315, and 345 degrees radially around the point of fixation. The average normal visual field score is 100; a score of 20 or less corresponds to an impairment rating of 80 percent or more.

According to the *Guides*, tangent screen testing and confrontation testing are insufficient for assessing permanent impairment. These methods involve the manual movement of a disc against a physical background or of the physician's finger in the air. Instead, it is suggested that examiners use either a Goldmann manual kinetic perimeter with the III/4e isopter or semiautomated kinetic perimetry with an equivalent "pseudoisopter"; this guidance is in line with SSA's perimetry requirements, which are mentioned specifically in the *Guides*.

The *Guides* require manual or semiautomated kinetic perimetry for visual field assessment. The text notes that most static methods measure only the central 30 degrees of the visual field—that is, 30 degrees from the point of central fixation—and are therefore insufficient for the functional assessment of visual field loss, which requires measurement out to a 60-degree radius. If only larger isopters are available, they may be used with the understanding that they may underestimate field loss. Since smaller isopters would overestimate field loss, they are deemed unacceptable for impairment evaluation.

Many states also use various editions of the AMA *Guides* for assessing impairment in their own workers' compensation programs (LexisNexis, 2019). However, some use their own state-developed standards. For example, New York State's *Workers' Compensation Guidelines for Determining Impairment* (Workers' Compensation Board, 2017, p. 60) require that visual field extent be measured using "a perimetric method with a white target." Like the *Guides*, the New York State *Guidelines* state that this method should be either a manual Goldmann kinetic perimeter with the III/4e isopter or an equivalent automated perimeter.

Federal Employees Retirement System

Another program for federal workers, the Federal Employees Retirement System (FERS), also offers disability retirement for civil servants who become disabled in a way that precludes "useful and efficient service" in their current or similar roles.[4] Chapter 60 of the Civil Service Retirement

---

[4] See 5 CFR § 844.102 "Useful and efficient service."

System and FERS *Handbook*, which describes requirements and procedures for these disability annuities, include "Job Aids" that guide examining physicians in providing acceptable medical evidence (U.S. Office of Personnel Management, 1998). Section 60C1.1-10 contains such guidance for eye disorders. This section of the *Handbook* advises that confrontation testing is useful as a base physical examination and that perimetry may be useful as a "special study." However, it does not require any specific perimeter or methodology.

Railroad Retirement Board

Retired railroad workers often receive a Railroad pension instead of Social Security retirement benefits. Railroad retirement benefits include a disability benefit. The Railroad Retirement Board (RRB), which manages retirement benefits for railroad workers, also manages disability evaluations and commensurate benefits. Generally, RRB impairment evaluations align with SSA's Listing of Impairments, and while SSA disability determinations are not binding on RRB decisions, they are part of the evidence that RRB considers.[5]

However, the RRB also maintains its own *Disability Claims Manual* (*DCM*), which is used primarily to determine whether a person's disability fully precludes them from railroad work as opposed to any regular work.[6] The *DCM* prefers that visual field testing be performed using an arc perimetry device (RRB, 2021). Arc perimetry, which is typically fully manual and does not use computerized measurement, involves the movement of a disc along an arc-shaped track. This arc can be rotated to test along different angles. The device should use a 3-millimeter white disc-shaped target set at a distance of 330 millimeters from the examinee, and illumination for the test should be at least 7 foot-candles. However, a handheld arc perimeter (essentially a handheld disc) or a traditional (manual) Goldmann kinetic perimeter is also acceptable. The *DCM* further states that tangent screening and "various automated perimeters" are "not desirable instruments for disability determination purposes" because such devices "record an erroneously more constricted" visual field than the permitted perimeters (RRB, 2021, p. 65).

EMPLOYMENT QUALIFICATIONS

Other agencies assess visual field extent to determine eligibility for employment in roles requiring good vision. Such eligibility requirements will often define an acceptable range for visual field extent and may or

---

[5] See 20 CFR § 220.100(b)(3) and 74 FR 63598.

[6] See 20 CFR § 220.10(a). Typically, disabilities precluding *any* work will be evaluated using SSA's listings and methodology for the purposes of RRB disability annuities.

may not define a preferred method for measurement. These requirements differ from SSA's disability requirements in that they are designed to assess suitability for a specific occupation, whereas SSA's disability determination process is meant to assess a person's ability to hold *any* gainful occupation.

Federal Aviation Administration

The Federal Aviation Administration (FAA) requires that pilots obtain a medical certificate before flying. Different types of pilots need different classes of certificates. First- and second-class medical certificates, which are, respectively, necessary for airline transport pilots and other commercial pilots, require normal fields of vision.[7] Air traffic controllers must also hold a second-class medical certificate.[8]

FAA medical certificates are granted by designated aviation medical examiners. Item 53 in the FAA's (2025) *Guide for Aviation Medical Examiners* describes how aviation medical examiners test fields of vision. The FAA prefers a tangent screen test using a 2-millimeter white test object on a black-handled holder against a 50-square-inch black matte wall target. For this method, results are recorded as the distance from the fixation point, in inches, at which the examinee first identifies the target object along each radial. However, a "standard perimeter" or confrontation test is also permitted, although the *Guide* advises that confrontation tests vision primarily at the periphery rather than centrally. If a perimeter is used, "any significant deviation from normal field configuration will require evaluation by an eye specialist" (FAA, 2025, p. 393). No specific perimeter is mentioned as required.

Federal Railroad Administration

While the vast majority of railroads in the United States are privately owned and operated, the Federal Railroad Administration (FRA) requires that conductors and locomotive engineers have a "field of vision of at least 70 degrees in the horizontal meridian [or diameter] of each eye."[9]

Beyond FRA requirements, individual railroads are given discretion to design their preferred medical assessments. As of 2018, for example, Union

---

[7] See 14 CFR § 67.103(d) and 14 CFR § 67.203(d).

[8] See 14 CFR § 65.31(c).

[9] See 49 CFR § 240.121(c)(2) and 49 CFR § 242.117(h)(2). In the literature and in this report, *meridian* typically refers to a line from the fixation point to the edge of the visual field (i.e., a radius). While FRA's requirements do not specify its meaning, typically the term *horizontal meridian* refers in the literature to a line running from the edge of the visual field nasally, through the fixation point, and to the other edge temporally (i.e., a diameter).

Pacific Railroad (2018) allowed for the use of automated perimeters such as the Humphrey Field Analyzer static automated perimeter, as well as Goldmann manual kinetic perimetry, when needed to measure full visual fields. A 2015 interim rule interpretation from FRA clarified that "the railroad must be able to cite a rigorous scientific study published in a peer-reviewed scientific or medical publication that demonstrates the scientific test is a valid, reliable, and comparable test for that visual capacity."[10] This differs from SSA guidelines, which require three clinical validation studies.

Federal Motor Carrier Safety Administration

The Federal Motor Carrier Safety Administration (FMCSA) sets regulations for drivers of commercial motor vehicles (e.g., truck drivers), such as physical qualifications. Like the FAA, FMCSA employs approved medical examiners to provide physical certification. Drivers must generally have a field of vision of at least 70 degrees horizontally in both eyes.[11] Use of a specific measurement methodology is not required.

If only one eye fails to meet this standard, applicants may meet an alternative vision standard instead.[12] Under this standard, both eyes must be retested, and the better eye must be verified to meet the 70-degree requirement. For this retest only, FMCSA mandates that an applicant's visual field be tested out to 120 degrees horizontally (i.e., 60 degrees both temporally and nasally). No specific type of perimetry or perimeter is mandated.

Other Federal Agencies

Several other federal visual field standards for hiring are listed below. Note that these agencies do not require that any specific test be performed, and each specifies a total visual field extent across the combined nasal and temporal meridians:

- *U.S. Merchant Mariner Medical Manual*: Requires that "the horizontal field of vision should not be less than 100 degrees in each eye" for deck personnel and other crew, such as engineers, tankermen, barge supervisors, and radio officers (USCG, 2019, pp. 5-1, 5-2).
- Federal Interagency Wildland Firefighter Medical Standards: Require "peripheral vision of at least 85 [degrees] laterally in each eye" for wildland firefighters, "which is generally considered to be normal" (USDA, n.d., p. 5).

---

[10] See 80 FR 73122.
[11] See 49 CFR § 391.41(b)(10)(i). See earlier footnote on the term "horizontal meridian."
[12] See 49 CFR § 391.44.

- Commissioned Corps of the U.S. Public Health Service Medical Accession Standards (USPHS, 2022): Require at least "30 degrees in either eye; a continuous field of vision which is [at least] 140 degrees (testing both eyes together)" for both Active Duty and Ready Reserve Corps members (p. 9).

The variation in these requirements suggests that, at least occupationally, the bar for meaningful visual impairment is vocation specific.

FUNCTIONAL CRITERIA

Some federal programs define visual impairment or disability according to functional criteria. Methods for measuring and systematically defining functional vision are well documented in the literature (Colenbrander, 2010; Massof, 2022). However, federal programs using such criteria tend to leave room for broader judgment based on the visual field extent necessary for normal activities. Such definitions are most commonly seen in federal accessibility rules.

Department of Education

The Department of Education's Office of Special Education Programs (OSEP) oversees the efforts of state and local education agencies to make education accessible for children with disabilities. These activities are authorized and regulated by the Individuals with Disabilities Education Act (IDEA). IDEA lists disabilities that make students eligible for special education services[13]; state and local education agencies must evaluate students according to these federal guidelines.[14]

On May 22, 2017, OSEP (2017) offered guidance to state and local education agencies on appropriate procedures for evaluating visual impairment. This guidance noted that for some disabilities, agencies have discretion to define certain qualifiers found in federal law. An example of an IDEA definition with such a qualifier is *orthopedic impairment*, defined as "a severe orthopedic impairment that adversely affects a child's educational performance."[15] While state and local standards may not be narrower than the definitions laid out in IDEA, agencies would be allowed, in this instance, to determine what qualifies as a "severe" impairment. However, the OSEP guidance noted that IDEA's definition of visual impairment does not include a modifier such as *severe*

---
[13] See 34 CFR § 300.8.
[14] See 34 CFR § 300.122.
[15] See 34 CFR § 300.8(c)(8).

that could be open to interpretation. IDEA defines *visual impairment including blindness* as "an impairment in vision that, even with correction, adversely affects a child's educational performance."[16] According to OSEP's (2017) interpretation, this means that *any* visual impairment that adversely affects a student's educational performance must qualify that student for special education services "regardless of significance or severity." OSEP (2017) further advised that basing eligibility for special education solely on specific diagnostic criteria without considering the degree to which the student's vision affects their educational performance is "inconsistent with the IDEA." Instead, agencies must use a holistic approach that considers educational, behavioral, medical, and other factors to determine how a child's visual impairment affects them in the classroom.

Statutes governing specific Department of Education programs are written similarly, operationalizing functional criteria. One such program assists state and local education agencies in providing accessible instructional materials for students with disabilities. Agencies must meet certain requirements to remain eligible for this assistance, including aligning their definitions for impairments with federal standards. To be an "eligible person"[17] who may receive services from these programs, a student may either meet the federal definition of statutory blindness or meet criteria related to their ability to access standard educational materials.

Federal law outlines two such functional criteria, either of which is sufficient for a student's eligibility[18]:

- The individual "has a visual impairment or perceptual or reading disability that cannot be improved to give visual function substantially equivalent to that of a person who has no such impairment or disability and so is unable to read printed works to substantially the same degree as a person without an impairment or disability;" or
- The individual "is otherwise unable, through physical disability, to hold or manipulate a book or to focus or move the eyes to the extent that would be normally acceptable for reading."

Eligibility must be confirmed by one of a list of approved medical or educational experts who use their professional judgment to assess how students' impairments will affect their ability to learn. No specific measurement or diagnosis is required.

---

[16] See 34 CFR § 300.8(c)(13).
[17] See 2 U.S. Code § 135a.
[18] See 2 USC § 135a(g)(1) and 17 USC § 121(d)(3).

Equal Employment Opportunity Commission

The Equal Employment Opportunity Commission (EEOC) takes an approach similar to the of the Department of Education in enforcing the employment provisions of the Americans with Disabilities Act (ADA). Under the ADA, an impairment qualifies as a disability if it substantially limits major life activities; federal law further provides that the phrase "substantially limit" should be interpreted as broadly as possible.[19]

In a 2023 guidance document, EEOC (2023) further noted that, given federal law, visual impairments do not need to prevent or severely restrict vision in order to quality as a disability. The use of mitigation measures other than ordinary glasses or contacts, such as low-vision devices, to improve a person's vision does not disqualify a person from disability protections. In general, EEOC considers visual impairments as disabilities based not on specific diagnosis but on their impacts on day-to-day life. While SSA does include functional assessment in later steps of its disability determination process (see Chapter 1), agencies such as EEOC differ by referring only to effects on an individual's functioning.

SUMMARY AND CONCLUSION

As described in Chapter 1, SSA outlines specific requirements for visual field testing to inform disability determinations. The guidelines clarify when and how different methods, such as static automated threshold perimetry and manual or semiautomated kinetic perimetry, are to be used, ensuring that test results align with SSA standards. Like SSA, many other government agencies have their own definitions of disability and visual impairment and their accepted methods for assessing visual field loss. These assessments are used to determine eligibility for disability benefits, eligibility for other disability-related programs, or qualification for jobs. Most go beyond the federal definition of statutory blindness, which requires that the widest diameter of a person's visual field be 20 degrees or less. Some agencies, similar to SSA, use statutory blindness as one of several medical criteria a person can meet to qualify as having a disability. Others adopt a functional definition of visual impairment, based on potential obstacles to engaging in relevant daily tasks. Most, however, set a specific visual field size that examinees must meet or not meet. The preferred perimeters and measurement techniques also differ among agencies, with some permitting a broader selection than others.

Some agencies assess visual field extent to determine eligibility for employment in roles requiring good vision. For example, the FAA requires

---

[19] See 29 CFR § 1630.2(j)(1)(i).

that pilots obtain a medical certificate before flying, and FRA requires that conductors and locomotive engineers have a "field of vision of at least 70 degrees in the horizontal [diameter] of each eye."[20] Varied requirements in occupationally based visual assessment suggest that the bar for meaningful visual impairment is vocation specific.

Other federal programs define visual impairment or disability based on functional criteria rather than specific diagnostic measures, emphasizing the impact on activities such as education or daily living. The Department of Education's OSEP, under IDEA, requires a holistic evaluation of how visual impairments affect a child's educational performance, ensuring eligibility for special education services regardless of severity. Federal accessibility programs similarly define eligibility using functional criteria, such as the inability to access standard educational materials, as verified by qualified experts. EEOC, under the Americans with Disabilities Act, adopts a broad interpretation of disability, focusing on how impairments limit major life activities rather than on specific diagnoses or severity.[21] This approach highlights the emphasis on functional impact over the type of objective medical criteria found in federal disability evaluations.

Based on its review of the literature, the committee reached the following conclusion:

Conclusion 2.1: Different federal government agencies have their own definitions of disability and visual impairment and their accepted methods for assessing visual field loss for a variety of purposes, including determining eligibility for disability benefits, eligibility for other disability-related programs, or qualification for certain jobs.

REFERENCES

AMA (American Medical Association). 2024. *AMA guides to the evaluation of permanent impairment*, 6th ed.

Colenbrander, A. 2010. Assessment of functional vision and its rehabilitation. *Acta Ophthalmologica* 88(2):163–173.

EEOC (U.S. Equal Employment Opportunity Commission). 2023. *Visual disabilities in the workplace and the Americans with Disabilities Act*. https://www.eeoc.gov/laws/guidance/visual-disabilities-workplace-and-americans-disabilities-act (accessed February 3, 2025).

FAA (Federal Aviation Administration). 2025. *Guide for aviation medical examiners*. https://www.faa.gov/ame_guide/media/ame_guide.pdf (accessed February 3, 2025).

LexisNexis. 2019. *State-by-state use of AMA guides*. https://www.lexisnexis.com/LegalNewsRoom/cfs-file/__key/telligent-evolution-components-attachments/01-221-00-00-01-44-08-54/AMAGuidesStatebyState.pdf (accessed April 21, 2025).

---

[20] See 49 CFR § 240.121(c)(2).
[21] See 29 CFR § 1630.2(j)(1)(i).

Massof, R. W. 2022. Patient-reported measures of the effects of vision impairments and low vision rehabilitation on functioning in daily life. *Annual Review of Vision Science* 8:217–238.

OSEP (Office of Special Education Programs). 2017. *Memorandum: Eligibility determinations for children suspected of having a visual impairment including blindness under the Individuals with Disability Education Act.* U.S. Department of Education. https://sites.ed.gov/idea/files/letter-on-visual-impairment-5-22-17.pdf (accessed February 3, 2025).

RRB (U.S. Railroad Retirement Board). 2021. *Disability claims manual part 4 medical evidence development and evaluation.* https://www.rrb.gov/sites/default/files/2022-12/DCM_Part_4_0.pdf (accessed February 3, 2025).

Union Pacific Railroad. 2018. *Medical standards for safety critical workers.* https://www.up.com/cs/groups/public/@uprr/@employee/@hr/documents/up_pdf_nativedocs/cdf_up_hr_hms_med_stnrds_visio.pdf (accessed February 4, 2025).

U.S. Office of Personnel Management. 1998. Chapter 60. Disability retirement. In *Civil Service Retirement System (CSRS) and Federal Employees Retirement System (FERS) handbook for personnel and payroll offices.* https://www.opm.gov/retirement-center/publications-forms/csrsfers-handbook/c060.pdf (accessed April 21, 2025).

USCG (U.S. Coast Guard). 2019. *Merchant mariner medical manual.* https://media.defense.gov/2019/Sep/11/2002181050/-1/-1/0/CIM_16721_48.pdf (accessed February 3, 2025).

USDA (U.S. Department of Agriculture). n.d. *Federal interagency wildland firefighter medical standards.* https://www.fs.usda.gov/sites/default/files/federal-interagency-wildland-firefighter-medical-standards.pdf (accessed February 3, 2025).

USPHS (Commissioned Corps of the U.S. Public Health Service). 2022. *CCI 221.01. Medical accession standards.* https://www.usphs.gov/media/4nhfmjln/medical-accession-standards-tab-a.pdf (accessed January 28, 2025).

Workers' Compensation Board. 2017. *Worker's compensation guidelines for determining impairment.* New York State of Opportunity. https://www.wcb.ny.gov/2018-Impairment-Guidelines.pdf (accessed February 3, 2025).

3

Current and Emerging Practice in Visual Field Testing

Perimetry, also known as visual field testing, is an essential diagnostic tool for assessing various ophthalmic conditions, including glaucoma, optic neuropathies, and disorders affecting the retina and visual pathways. Box 3-1 depicts some types of field losses associated with different ophthalmic conditions. Static automated threshold perimetry (SAP), also commonly referred to as standard automated perimetry, measures the sensitivity of an individual's visual field at specific test locations (within 10, 24, or 30 degrees from the point of central fixation[1] depending on the testing pattern employed) and has the capability to compare the findings with a database of previously tested patients with normal vision. SAP employs white stimuli against white backgrounds and is valuable not only for initial diagnosis but also for monitoring disease progression and guiding treatment decisions (Ruia and Tripathy, 2023). In glaucoma care, SAP is the primary method used to assess visual field loss and monitor changes over time (AAO, 2020; AOA, 2024).

In this report, perimetry refers to the general technique of measuring visual fields by mapping threshold sensitivities in the central and peripheral fields. Perimetry utilizes a variety of specific instruments and testing protocols, including the most recognizable and conventional methods—Humphrey static automated perimetry and Goldmann manual kinetic perimetry—in addition to newer methods using novel display types, such as head-mounted virtual reality displays. In addition, optokinetic perimetry holds promise for assessing

---

[1] Point of central fixation or central fixation refers to the point where an examinee focuses their gaze during a visual field test, essentially serving as the center and reference point for mapping the extent and sensitivity of the visual field.

BOX 3-1
Types of Visual Field Losses

A variety of ophthalmic conditions can cause different types of visual field impairment, as illustrated in Figure 3-1 below. Glaucoma can lead to tunnel vision, which worsens as the condition progresses, as shown in Panel B. Glaucoma can also result in one or more typically arcuate scotomas (an area within the visual field in which stimuli are not seen at an intensity expected in that location, resulting in areas of blurry vision), and diabetic retinopathy can result in multiple scotomas, as shown in Panel C. Damage to the visual cortex on one side of the brain, such as from a stroke or head injury, can result in hemianopia, which is the loss of half the visual field, as shown in Panels D1 and D2. These panels depict different examples of hemianopia for a single eye. In D1, the affected half of the field is still visible but is very blurry; in D2, the affected left half of the field is entirely absent. Advanced age-related macular degeneration can result in a blurry area in the center of the visual field, as shown in (Panel E).

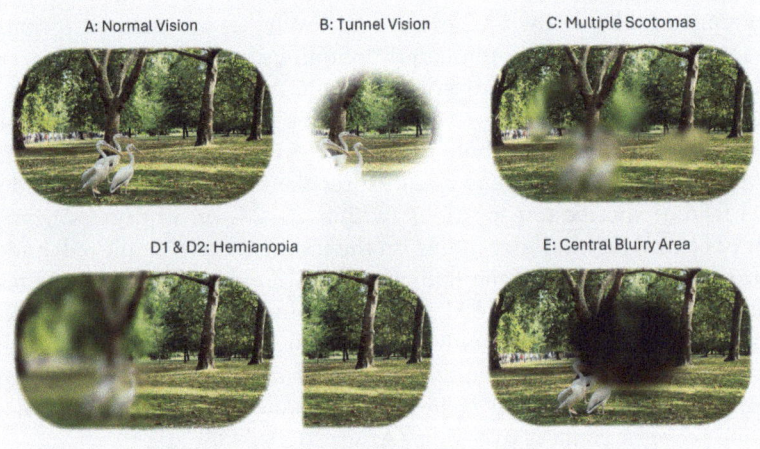

FIGURE 3-1 Simulation of selected types of visual field losses.
Photo credit: Tina M. Winters.

individuals who are unable to maintain fixation on a central location. This chapter presents an overview of the fundamentals of perimetry and the current practice landscape for the measurement of visual field impairment with perimetry devices, describes recent changes and challenges in the provision of such care, and provides a summary of emerging perimetry technologies.

FUNDAMENTALS OF PERIMETRY

The visual field is the extent of an area visible to an individual during steady fixation of the eye in any one gaze or direction. It can be pictured as a "hill of vision" (see Figure 3-1), a concept first introduced by Harry Traquair (1947, p. 4) that represents the visual field as a "hill of vision surrounded by a sea of blindness." Retinal sensitivity is highest at the fovea and deceases toward the periphery (Ruia and Tripathy, 2023; Weber and Caprioli, 2000). This concept is represented in perimetry output as a central peak in sensitivity at the fixation point, with sensitivity gradually decreasing in all directions. Loci of equal sensitivity on this surface form isosensitivity contours (isopters), analogous to contour lines on a topographic map or isobars on a meteorological map. Closely spaced isopters indicate a steep slope in visual sensitivity, while widely spaced ones reflect a gentler slope. At the outermost edge of the visual field, the island of vision descends into a "sea of blindness," signifying a complete lack of perception beyond the peripheral boundary (Schiefer et al., 2005). Temporally, or at the outer boundaries of the visual field toward the temple, the slope is less steep compared with the region immediately surrounding the fovea (see Figure 3-2).

The Social Security Administration (SSA) considers the normal visual field to extend approximately 60 degrees nasally (toward the nose) and inferiorly (downward), 45 degrees superiorly (upward), and 85 degrees

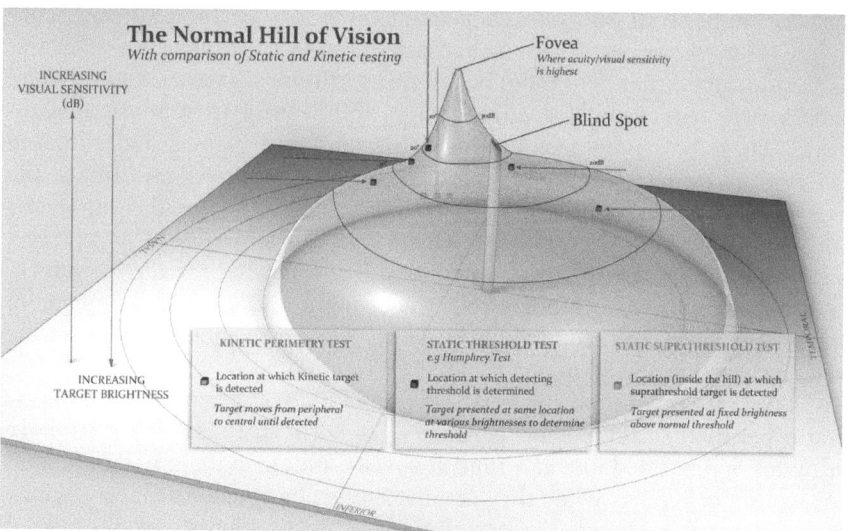

FIGURE 3-2 Normal hill of vision for a right eye.
SOURCE: Wong and Plant (2015), reproduced with permission from BMJ Publishing Group Ltd.

temporally (in the opposite direction from the nose) (SSA, n.d.-a [Listings], Figure 1; see also footnote 3 in Chapter 5). The standard unit for measuring the visual field is differential light sensitivity, which defines the threshold for detecting a test object relative to its background, also known as the surround. Visual sensitivity is expressed in decibels (dB), which is a logarithmic unit. As discussed below, a larger value for the number of decibels (e.g., 35 dB vs. 15 dB) indicates greater attenuation of the stimulus and corresponds to increased visual sensitivity.

Decibels, a relative logarithmic unit of attenuation, rather than objective units of luminosity, are used because of Weber's law. Weber's law states that the change in light intensity required to elicit a noticeable response from the visual system is proportional to the previous light intensity. Mathematically speaking, this means that the patient's perception of contrast during perimetry is proportional to the logarithm of the difference in intensity between the stimulus and the background. As a result, visual sensitivity is usually reported on a decibel scale. It is similar to the use of decibels to report sound intensities; sounds, like visual stimuli, are perceived as sensory signals that differ in intensity from one another. The law holds closely at normal daylight levels (known as photopic light levels) but breaks down at twilight (mesopic) and low light (scotopic) levels.

With age, visual field sensitivities and limits decline (Weber and Caprioli, 2000), illustrating the importance of normative databases that represent the full range of age and other demographic characteristics. Normative data may or may not be stratified by age, depending on which data point is being considered. Acuity norms are not age adjusted, but visual field sensitivities are.

A normal visual field relies on several anatomical factors: clear optical media, proper focus of the retinal image, and healthy afferent visual pathways. These pathways include photoreceptors and bipolar and ganglion cells in the retina, ganglion cell axons in the optic nerves and tracts, the lateral geniculate body, the optic radiations, and the neuronal components of the primary visual cortex (Schiefer et al., 2005). Figure 3-3 depicts a simplified graphic of this pathway. Note, however, that the direct connection depicted between bipolar cells and ganglion cells does not occur in mammalian eyes; instead, there are other types of cells such as AII amacrine cells involved in this pathway (Kolb, 1995).

There are two broad categories of perimetry in conventional use today: static perimetry and kinetic perimetry. In static perimetry, a stationary stimulus is presented one at a time at specific points in the visual field, and the examinee reports when they see a stimulus. In kinetic perimetry, which can be manual, automated, or semiautomated, a stimulus is typically moved from a nonseeing to a seeing area with the patient reporting when they first see it. Both are commonly conducted using a hemispherical surface onto which the visual field is mapped (see Figure 3-4). The examined eye is positioned near the geometric center of the hemisphere, ensuring that

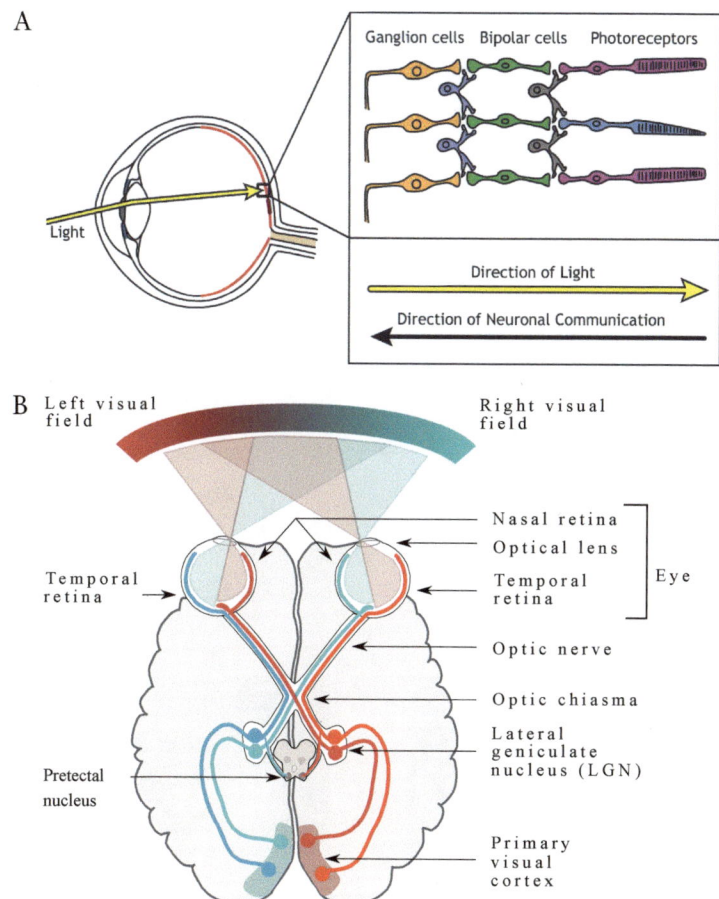

FIGURE 3-3 The human visual pathway.
SOURCE: Panel A: Henley (2021). CC BY-NC-SA 4.0; Panel B: Nieto (2015). CC BY SA 4.0.

all points on the inner surface of the hemisphere are equidistant from the eye. The examinee is instructed to maintain their gaze on a central fixation point throughout the test.[2] The surface is evenly illuminated, and test objects consist of small light spots projected onto that background (termed the surround; Schiefer et al., 2005).

In practical application, the background brightness (luminance) is kept constant while a test object (stimulus point of light) of varying size, brightness, and position is projected onto it. This can be done by moving the test

---

[2] Many perimeters offer the option of four points in a diamond format to allow individuals with central scotomata to maintain fixation.

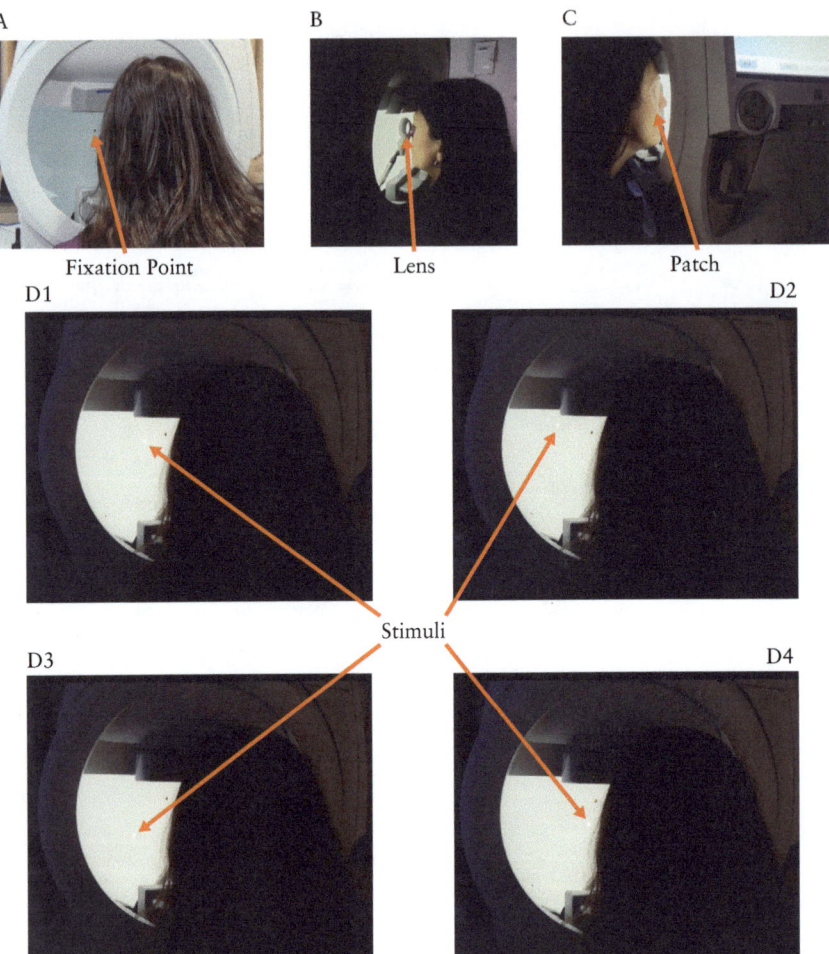

FIGURE 3-4 Static automated threshold perimetry testing experience.
Photo credit: Tina M. Winters.
NOTE: This figure illustrates various components of static visual field testing conducted in a bowl perimetry device. The patient is instructed to maintain their gaze on a central fixation point, as shown in Panel A. Once the head is positioned correctly for the test, the lights are dimmed in the room, as shown in the subsequent panels. Each eye is tested individually; a lens is placed in front of the tested eye (Panel B), and the eye that is not undergoing testing is occluded with a patch (Panel C). Once the test begins, a series of stimuli (white lights) are projected onto the surface of the bowl (Panels D1–D4), and the patient is instructed to press a button each time they see a stimulus.

object with constant size and brightness (kinetic perimetry) or by projecting stationary stimuli one at a time at different locations on the background (static perimetry). Static threshold perimetry involves maintaining the same stimulus size and/or brightness throughout the test or adjusting the size and/ or brightness over the course of the test. The threshold is probabilistically determined as the intensity or contrast that results in a 50 percent likelihood of detecting the object at a specific location within the visual field. The boundary of the visual field is considered the point in the visual field that separates the area that is seen from that which is not seen. If there is an area that falls within the boundary of the visual field in which stimuli are not seen at an intensity expected in that location, this area is referred to as a scotoma. A blind spot is an area in which a stimulus is not seen at any intensity.

As shown in Figure 3-2, normal vision includes a physiological blind spot, which corresponds to the location of the optic nerve where there is no visual sensitivity. Most diagnostic tests focus on the area within 30 degrees of central fixation because the greatest concentration of retinal ganglion cells is located in this area. The area beyond 30 degrees is considered part of the peripheral visual field, where there is greater variation in the measurement of visual sensitivity.

Perimetry testing employs standardized stimulus sizes developed by Goldmann (Figure 3-5). To determine visual sensitivity in static automated

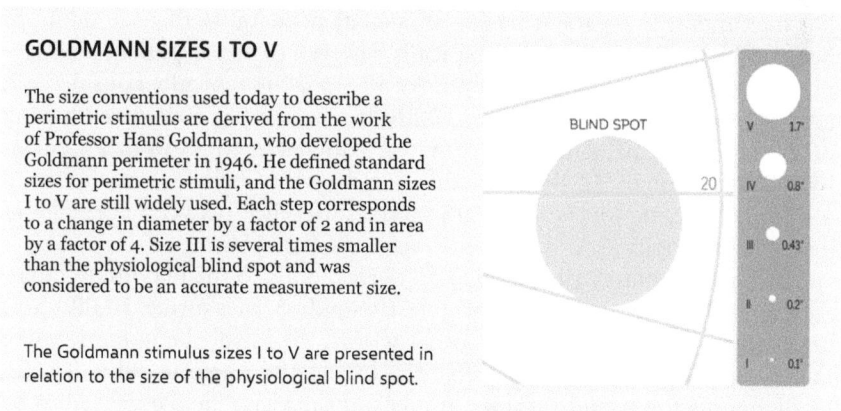

FIGURE 3-5 Goldmann stimulus sizes.
NOTE: The figure depicts the five stimulus sizes developed by Goldmann that are typically employed in perimetry, as compared with the size of the physiological blind spot. To illustrate in practical terms, Goldmann size III approximately corresponds to the size of the full moon in the sky.
SOURCE: Racette et al. (2019). Copyright © HAAG-STREIT AG.

threshold perimetry, the stimulus intensity is varied at static locations. The Humphrey static automated perimeter is capable of projecting stimuli at various intensities in Goldmann stimulus sizes of I, II, III, IV, and V— corresponding to 0.1 degree, 0.21 degree, 0.43 degree, 0.86 degree, and 1.72 degrees in diameter, respectively. While these are often used to correspond to different sizes apparent to the viewer (i.e., the Goldmann III-4e stimulus corresponding to an area of 4 mm^2), people whose eyes have different axial lengths can technically perceive slightly different sizes of stimulus. The diameter of the stimulus on the perimeter's bowl is fixed, but only for a similar bowl size; a 0.43-degree stimulus for the size III stimulus is the same no matter the bowl's make. The Goldmann size III (0.43 degree) is most commonly used. The background illumination within the Humphrey device is uniformly set at 10 candelas per square meter (31.4 apostilbs [asb]), the level originally used in the Goldmann manual kinetic perimeter, reviewed later in this chapter. This level of illumination is thought to be less affected than other levels by change in the size of the pupil or existing lens opacification and is within the range at which Weber's law still applies. The Humphrey perimeter projects light stimuli ranging from 0.1 to 10,000 asb or 0.03 to 3,183 candelas per square meter.

As stated, decibels are a logarithmic measurement of the attenuation of a stimulus compared to the maximum available. The contrast presented is the stimulus luminance divided by the background luminance. Thus, in perimetry, a 0-dB stimulus refers to the highest contrast stimulus that the device can present, and a 30-dB stimulus has 3 log-units lower contrast than that maximum. If a patient has a 50 percent probability of responding to the 30-dB stimulus, then that is typically referred to as the patient having a sensitivity of 30 dB at that location. As 30–35 dB is typically considered a normal level of sensitivity, having 10 dB of sensitivity is considered having 20–25 dB of impairment, approximately equivalent to SSA's mean deviation requirement of 22 dB to qualify for disability benefits. As discussed in Chapter 1, mean deviation averages the difference between normal and observed sensitivities.

On the Humphrey perimeter, 0 dB corresponds to the maximum intensity the perimeter can present (brightest stimulus), measuring 10,000 asb; 50 dB corresponds to 0.1 asb. In other words, the lower the numeric value for dB, the brighter is the stimulus; the higher the numeric value for dB, the dimmer is the stimulus. Thus, at areas of the visual field expected to be most sensitive (i.e., the center), the visible dB range is expected to be at its highest (i.e., the dimmest stimuli can be perceived). The maximum stimulus sensitivity that would be expected in a normal individual is 40 dB (Heijl et al., 2021).

Static threshold perimetry, in which threshold sensitivities are mapped at predefined, static locations, can be either manual or automated, although manual static threshold perimetry, in which a technician manually presents the stimulus and records the examinee's responses, is rarely used today. In static automated threshold perimetry, test objects are presented across an area of the visual field, typically in a rectilinear grid, and a computer algorithm controls their display, minimizing examiner input. This approach allows for more efficient and consistent testing. By interpolating the differential light sensitivity values, this method generates a graphic representation of the hill of vision, resembling the polygonal facets of a geodesic dome (Schiefer et al., 2005). An example of a Humphrey visual field test printout depicting this graphic representation is shown in Figure 3-6.

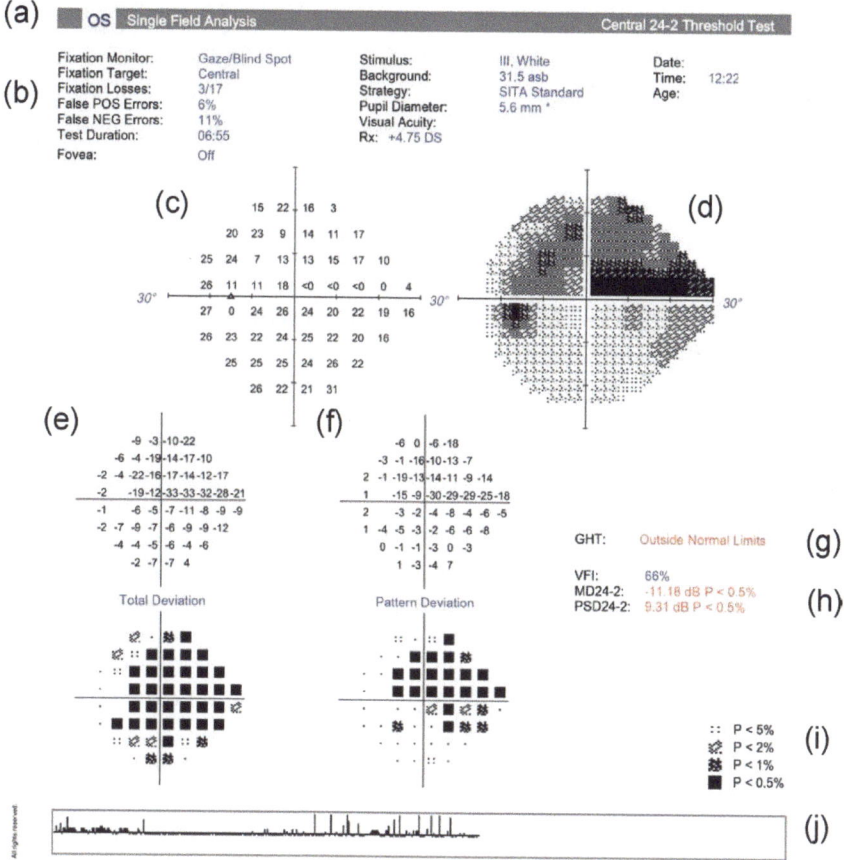

FIGURE 3-6 Humphrey visual field printout.
NOTES: asb = apostilb; dB = decibel; MD = mean deviation; OS = oculus sinister (left eye); p = probability; PSD = pattern standard deviation; VFI = visual field index.
SOURCE: Wu et al. (2022). Reprinted with permission from Elsevier.

Humphrey visual field static automated threshold perimetry provides a comprehensive review of an individual's visual field, yielding critical information that is useful in assessing performance, comparison with a normative database, and validity. The test printout in Figure 3-6 (a) specifies the test type and eye tested, in this case a 24-2 SITA[3] Standard Test single-field analysis of the left eye (*oculus sinister*). This individual's left eye demonstrates an advanced superior arcuate scotoma with split fixation and a nasal step. Figure 3-6 (b) shows that the fixation monitor was on during the test and that the fixation target was located centrally. It also specifies reliability indices, specifically fixation losses, false positives, and false negatives; the duration of the test; and the fact that foveal threshold testing was turned off (when turned on, this testing yields a metric that correlates with visual acuity and is useful in cases in which there may be nonorganic visual acuity loss). Figure 3-6 (c) shows the numeric results as a plot of sensitivities by location and measured in decibels, while Figure 3-6 (d) shows a grayscale illustration of the numeric results. Figure 3-6 (e) is a plot illustrating the deviation of the measured decibels from the expected age-adjusted levels of sensitivity relative to specific locations in the visual field and the test strategy used. Positive values denote points demonstrating better-than-normal sensitivity, while negative values represent worse-than-normal sensitivity.

The Humphrey visual field printout also provides additional statistical analysis measuring the likelihood that the observed sensitivity at a given location is likely to correspond to what was expected at that location. The results of this analysis are located below each of the numerical plots. Thus, what is illustrated is the probability according to the legend shown in Figure 3-6 (i). Deviations from expected values are highlighted when they are worse than those found in the bottom 5 percent, 2 percent, 1 percent, and 0.5 percent of normal subjects who are the same age as the patient. Figure 3-6 (f) is a plot illustrating the deviation, corrected for conditions such as a cataract, which may diffusely impact the visual field.

Figure 3-6 (g) provides the results of the Glaucoma Hemifield Test, which is based on an automated statistical analysis of patterns expected to be observed in glaucoma patients undergoing either the 24-2 or 30-2 test patterns (testing patterns are explained in the section below on current practice in perimetry assessment). Scoring differences in the upper hemifield divided into specific zones are compared with the mirror image of the same zone in the lower hemifield. In this example, the Glaucoma Hemifield Test is outside normal limits.

Figure 3-6 (h) includes the global indices of visual field index, mean deviation, and pattern standard deviation. For this test, the visual field index is 66 percent, the mean deviation is −11.18 dB, and the pattern standard

---

[3] SITA is the Swedish Interactive Thresholding Algorithm, explained later in this chapter.

deviation is −9.31 dB. Visual field index, which is less affected than mean deviation by conditions such as cataract and is considered to correspond to ganglion cell loss, is a useful metric in tracking disease progression. Mean deviation 24-2 is the average of the total deviation plotted in Figure 3-6 (e). Pattern standard deviation 24-2 peaks when there are moderate levels of localized field loss and should not be used to detect progression. As noted previously, Figure 3-6 (i) lists the probability symbols used in Figure 3-6 (e). Finally, Figure 3-6 (j) is the gaze index, which illustrates the variability in the eye gaze throughout the test. This metric is generated by a dual-variable tracker that measures gaze direction when a stimulus is projected. Taller spikes on the chart indicate periods when the patient's focus deviated from the central fixation point by 10 degrees or more, while smaller spikes indicate smaller fixation losses. This visual display of the patient's gaze is useful in educating individuals who are new to visual field testing about the importance of maintaining fixation throughout the test, an important lesson when additional testing is needed to confirm observed defects. In summary, the totality of the Humphrey visual field printout gives the clinician information that is important for assessing the patient's visual function and performance and that can be used to inform future testing if needed.

In contrast to manual and automated static threshold perimetry, manual and semiautomated[4] kinetic perimetry employ test objects that typically are moved from nonseeing to seeing areas of the visual field (movement in the opposite direction is possible as well and in fact can be used in conjunction with traditional kinetic perimetry to provide an average; see Chapter 5). Each isopter or island of vision can be mapped by testing variable target sizes and intensities using a moving stimulus.

The subject is asked to indicate when the moving light stimulus first becomes visible as it is presented from the periphery along different meridians (see Figure 3-7). Meridians refer to imaginary lines radiating from the central focus point, dividing the visual field into equal sections like pieces of a pie. Typically, the visual field is divided into eight equal sections, with the meridians intersecting at the central focus point. The meridians are labeled in degrees (0, 45, 90, 135, 180, 225, 270, 315, and 360), moving counterclockwise from the 3 o'clock position. The borders from not seeing to seeing at different meridians can then be connected to outline the isopter, or island of vision, using different stimuli. These stimuli are typically bright. As a result, impairments limited to dim stimuli may not be determinable using kinetic perimetry. However, individuals with such impairment are likely to qualify for Social Security Disability Insurance under a different pathway; this report is concerned with only those related to the extent of

---

[4] In this report, the term semiautomated rather than automated kinetic perimetry is used to highlight the role of the clinician.

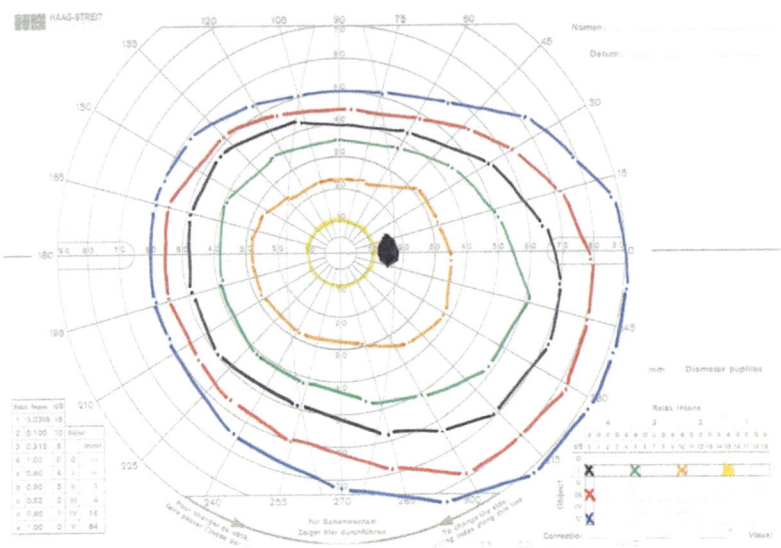

FIGURE 3-7 Example of Goldmann visual field plot.
SOURCE: Tahib et al. (2018). Reproduced with permission from Springer Nature.

the visual field as defined by SSA. It is important to map the physiological blind spot to ensure the validity of the test.

This approach has advantages over static perimetry, particularly (1) when there are more complex midperipheral or peripheral scotomas (e.g., a peripheral ring scotoma) associated with retinal or neuro-ophthalmic disease, (2) when the visual field status in the far periphery needs to be investigated, (3) when individuals have difficulty responding to the stimuli and the testing pace needs to be slower, and (4) with pediatric patients because of increased engagement. Overall, relative to static perimetry, results of kinetic perimetry provide a more functional perspective and snapshot of the total visual field present in the center and periphery, and in some ways a more thorough image of the morphology of complex scotomas since the isopter borders (islands of vision) are clearly defined.

Visual field efficiency is expressed as a percentage corresponding to the visual field in the better eye, calculated by summing the number of degrees seen along the eight principal meridians found on a visual field chart and dividing by 5. For example, if the visual field is contracted down to 25 degrees in all eight meridians, the remaining visual field efficiency is $25 \times 8 \div 5 = 40$ percent (SSA, n.d.-a, 2.00A7c).

There are also devices, such as the Octopus 900, that offer semiautomated kinetic perimetry testing. They are semiautomated because they combine manual and automated features; specifically, they allow for manual testing with customized testing patterns and focused area retesting, while controlling for the speed of kinetic stimulus presentation. Chapter 5 discusses the differences between automated and semiautomated perimetry in greater detail. When automated or semiautomated perimetry is not possible (or reliable), or when it is unavailable, other perimetry methods can be used, and their results may be analyzed together to gain a more holistic view of the total visual field function of the patient. For example, manual kinetic perimetry (or manual Goldmann perimetry) may be used along with alternative perimetry methods that may be more accessible, such as threshold frequency doubling technology (FDT). FDT uses a flickering stimulus to evaluate contrast sensitivity for specific stimuli. However, automated kinetic perimetry is commonly preferred to manual kinetic perimetry because it does not require access to trained personnel and offers the ability to standardize testing conditions (AAO, 2020; AOA, 2024; Ruia and Tripathy, 2023). FDT is discussed in greater detail in Chapter 5.

For individuals who may have a difficult time maintaining focus on a central location during the test, optokinetic perimetry may be considered rather than static threshold perimetry. Saccadic vector optokinetic perimetry (SVOP) is a novel modality for measuring visual fields, especially in younger children who cannot yet undergo quantitative visual field testing. SVOP is based on the principles of oculokinetic perimetry, a technique that provides a plotting of the visual field by having the patient move his or her eye, as described by Damato (1985), instead of presenting a static or kinetic stimulus while the patient maintains a fixed gaze and responds to stimuli based on predetermined locations. The SVOP test enables patients to respond to visual stimuli in a more natural and intuitive manner. Examinees need not focus on a specific location but instead have a response similar to that in electronic gaming. Since this technique tracks the eye position in three-dimensional space directly as it occurs throughout the testing, a more flexible testing environment is possible. Furthermore, a check is included in the SVOP system that halts the test when there is a conflict between the eye gaze data and the fixation stimuli coordinates. This allows for more accurate testing, and for a steadier interaction with visual stimuli and use of tracking in real time (Murray et al., 2009). Because of its benefit for examinees who have difficulty maintaining central fixation, this technology is theoretically beneficial for pediatric patients; however, this has not been clinically demonstrated as superior to current methods and so does not see widespread use in this population.

The visual field (the extent of an area visible to an individual during steady fixation of the eye in any one gaze or direction, as defined earlier) must be clearly distinguished from a person's ability to see the world around them in natural conditions when both the eyes and head can move. In everyday visual experience, these combined freedoms of movement increase total visual performance compared with the comparatively artificial concept of the visual field. In visual field testing, the diagnostic value of the data diminishes with increased degrees of movement because the performance of the ocular and somatic motor systems merges with that of the afferent sensory pathways. When movement is allowed, defects in the visual field can be concealed by compensatory movements of the eye, head, and/or body, potentially compromising the accuracy of the test results (Schiefer et al., 2005).

CURRENT PRACTICE IN PERIMETRY ASSESSMENT

Perimetry techniques include a combination of hardware, stimuli, testing patterns, and algorithms (Table 3-1). As discussed above, the stimulus is the visual signal presented during a visual field test, which can be static or kinetic. The technician administering the visual field test specifies the size of the stimulus (e.g., Goldmann size III, which has a diameter of 0.43 degree [Figure 3-5]) and the duration of the stimulus in milliseconds. Testing patterns are determined by the examiner based on clinical findings, diagnosis, and characteristics of the person being examined. The algorithm refers to the testing program, which is specific to the hardware. For example, the Humphrey Field Analyzer is generally paired with the Swedish Interactive Thresholding Algorithm (SITA).

Perimetry Hardware

Perimetry devices vary in design and portability, although the devices used most commonly tend to be large and not portable. Stimulus presentation varies across perimetry systems. While optical projection is standard, some devices now use LCD-based stimuli for consistent brightness and contrast. Sensitivity is measured in decibels, a logarithmic scale on which 0 dB represents the brightest light stimulus and 50 dB the dimmest. Knowing the brightness and luminance values of the stimulus and background of the perimeter is important for understanding the difference in dB scales among instruments when interpreting perimetry results.

The brightness capabilities of perimeters vary as well. In general, 0 dB reflects the machine's maximum brightness rather than a standard intensity. For the purpose of reporting, the results are often, but not always, normalized to reflect the results that would have been obtained from a Humphrey Field Analyzer (static automated threshold perimeter) when the same background level (10 candelas per square meter) is used. This statistical normalization, however, is only possible when the perimeter is operating within a luminance range for which Weber's law holds, and only under

TABLE 3-1 Field Testing Instruments, Testing Strategies, Testing Patterns, and Testing Algorithms

Instrument / Perimeter	Testing Strategies	Testing Patterns	Testing Algorithms	Comments
Humphrey Field Analyzer (HFA)	Static automated (Note: some models [HFA3 and HFA840-860] have kinetic testing ability)	30-2, 24-2, 10-2, 24-2C, 120-point (Esterman)	Swedish Interactive Thresholding Algorithm (SITA) Standard, SITA Fast, SITA Faster, Esterman screening (suprathreshold)	Widely used in the United States; measures central and peripheral fields; short-wavelength automated perimetry isolates short-wavelength cones for early glaucoma detection. Projected stimuli.
Octopus	Static automated and semiautomated kinetic	30-2, 24-2, 10-2, 60-4; G-program; M-Program; semiautomated kinetic testing	Full threshold, tendency-oriented perimetry, semiautomated kinetic algorithm	Common in Europe. Semiautomated kinetic testing provides controlled vector speed, reaction time compensation, and customizable templates for enhanced reliability. Projected stimuli.
Goldmann	Manual kinetic	Nonstandardized, technician dependent, manual testing pattern along principal meridians	[None]	Requires trained personnel. Projected stimuli.
Humphrey Matrix	Frequency doubling technology	N-20, C-30	Zippy Estimation by Sequential Testing (ZEST), screening	Evaluates visual function based on the individual's ability to detect a sinusoidal grating pattern (see Figure 5-1), but limited studies in severely affected individuals; portable device; testing can be performed in ambient lighting conditions.
imo Head-Mounted Perimeter	Static automated	30-2, 24-2, 10-2, 24-plus (78 points, including 24-2 and additional central points)	Ambient Interactive ZEST (AIZE)	Portable, uses head-mounted display; tests left and right eyes separately or binocularly; LCD screen.
Topcon Tempo	Standard automated	30-2, 24-2, 10-2, 24-plus	AIZE, AIZE-rapid, full threshold, two-zone (screening)	Desk-based version of imo; monocular or binocular testing; LCD screen.
iCare Compass	Fundus automated	30-2, 24-2, 10-2	ZEST, ZEST Rapid	Includes confocal retinal imaging and fixation tracking; LED screen.

NOTE: The imo, Tempo, and iCare Compass, as well as other virtual reality–based devices, are discussed in detail later in the chapter. See Table 5-1 in Chapter 5 for background and maximum luminance levels.

similar background luminance as the Humphrey Field Anaylzer. To ensure ongoing accuracy, the brightness of the stimulus must be calibrated either manually or automatically. Furthermore, in interpreting results, floor and ceiling effects relating to the machines' capabilities need to be considered.

Humphrey Field Analyzer

The Humphrey Field Analyzer is the static automated threshold perimeter that is currently most commonly used for visual field testing in the United States. It is especially prominent in detecting and monitoring glaucoma, given its ability to measure threshold sensitivities within the central and peripheral visual field; its reliability indices; and its specialized testing algorithms, such as SITA Standard, SITA Fast, and SITA Faster (Heijl et al., 2019; Ruia and Tripathy, 2023; Sikorsky and Laudencka, 2020). The Humphrey Field Analyzer offers 30-2, 24-2, 24-2C, and 10-2 testing patterns, allowing targeted assessment of the central visual field as well as more peripheral areas, which are essential for glaucoma and neuro-ophthalmologic assessments (AAO, 2020; AOA, 2024).

Octopus

The Octopus perimeter is also widely used, although it is more commonly used in Europe. It is valued for its flexibility, offering both static automated threshold and semiautomated kinetic testing options. It also employs unique algorithms, including the G-Program, which measures the sensitivity of a 30-degree field; the M-Program, which analyzes the macula area; and tendency-oriented perimetry for faster threshold testing. Octopus perimetry is often used for both general eye care and glaucoma follow-up, and it is compatible with various analysis programs, including glaucoma progression analyses and combined structure–function tests.

Goldmann

While no longer commercially available, the original Goldmann perimeter is a manual kinetic device still used by some clinicians. Because it is fully manual, it does not employ algorithms. A trained technician is needed to perform the test reliably, considering that various stimuli must be brought from the periphery to the center along a particular radian at a consistent speed. The technician must record reliably the point at which the patient first detects the stimulus. By repeating this maneuver at other angles of approach, a map of the visual field can be created. Usually, the technician will repeat a test once or twice using stimuli that require greater or lesser sensitivity. In addition to kinetic perimetric testing, the technician can test the patient's ability to detect specific stimuli centrally by projecting varying levels of stimulus luminosity.

Humphrey Matrix

The Humphrey Matrix evaluates contrast sensitivity using a sinusoidal flickering stimulus instead of a static circle, with available stimulus sizes of 2, 5, and 10 degrees. Testing with the Humphrey Matrix is faster but less comprehensive than testing with the Humphrey Field Analyzer and Octopus devices. Further discussion of the Humphrey Matrix, as well as frequency doubling technology in general, can be found in Chapter 5.

Testing Patterns and Strategies

In a perimetry test, the testing pattern refers to the set of points at which small lights are flashed at different intensities. As shown in Table 3-1, there are a number of testing patterns that may be employed. Testing patterns vary in the number of points and the span of the testing area. They are often noted in a #-# format, with the first # representing the extent of the field being tested in degrees, and the second # representing the specific pattern of points used during the test. For example, as shown in Figure 3-8, the 30-2 testing pattern extends 30 degrees from fixation and includes 76 points; the 24-2 testing pattern extends 24 degrees temporally and 30 degrees nasally from fixation and includes 54 points; and the 10-2 testing pattern extends only 10 degrees from fixation and includes 64 points. The 30-2 and 24-2 testing patterns present points 6 degrees apart, while the 10-2 program covers the central 10 degrees with higher resolution, presenting points spaced 2 degrees apart, and is thus better suited to detect early, subtle central defects. Recently, the 24-2C program introduced additional points within the central 10 degrees to improve the detection of paracentral scotomas, although it does not match the resolution of the 10-2 (Ruia and Tripathy, 2023).

Testing patterns can be tailored in response to the severity and location of visual field loss. For instance, central 10-degree testing patterns, such as the 10-2 test, are particularly valuable for patients with visual field damage that approaches fixation or for the detection of early central visual field defects that might not be identified by the 24-2 or 30-2 testing strategies (AAO, 2020). In such patients, focusing on the central 10 degrees using automated perimetry is useful, as it provides more sampling points close to this area than the 24-2, 24-2C, or 30-2 testing patterns. The examiner could use the 10-2 pattern for testing to identify early visual field loss in the central 10 degrees before such changes become apparent with more conventional larger-area test strategies, such as the 24-2 and 30-2 patterns.

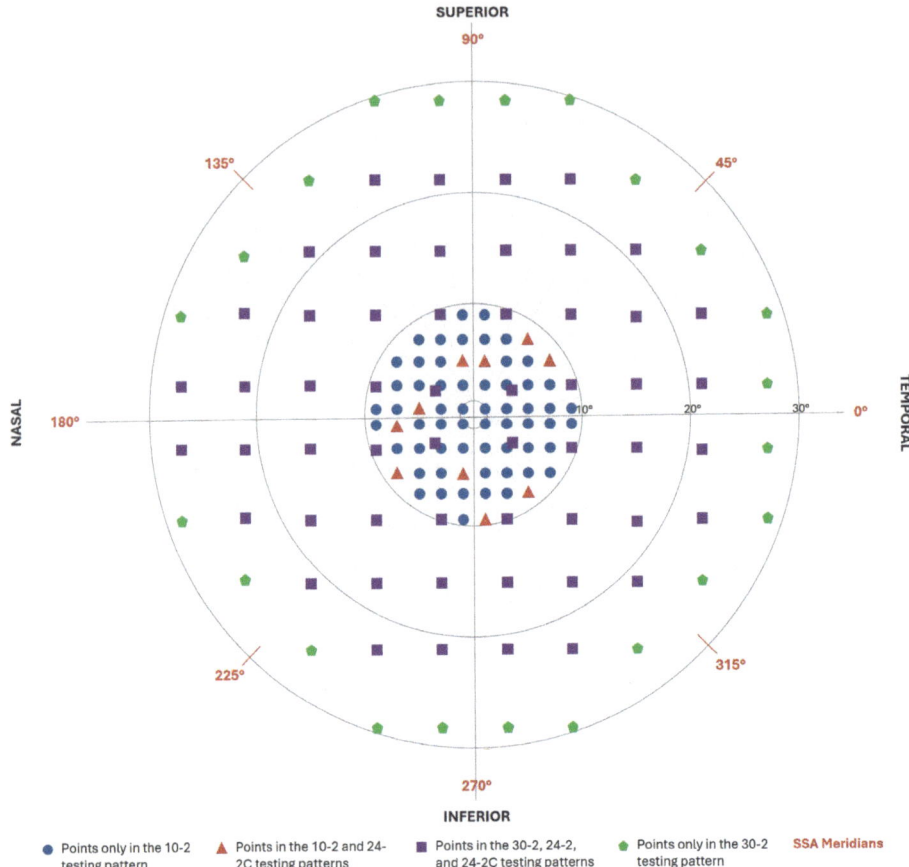

FIGURE 3-8 Examples of testing patterns (right eye).
NOTES: This figure illustrates the 10-2, 24-2, 24-2C, and 30-2 testing patterns available on the Humphrey Field Analyzer, showing approximate stimulus locations for each of these patterns. As illustrated, the 10-2 pattern presents stimulus points within 10 degrees of the fixation point, with the points beginning ±1 degree from central fixation. Points in the 10-2 pattern are separated by 2 degrees. The 24-2 and 30-2 patterns present stimulus points beginning ±3 degrees from central fixation, with points separated by 6 degrees. The 24-2 pattern includes 54 points, while the 30-2 pattern includes 76 points. The 24-C pattern includes all of the 54 points in the 24-2 pattern plus an additional 10 points within the central 10 degrees from fixation. The 10-2 pattern includes 68 points. The 24-2 and 24-2C testing patterns are differentiated by right eye and left eye; this figure depicts the patterns as they would be presented in testing for the right eye. SSA = Social Security Administration.

The committee notes that the 30-2 testing pattern is used less often in routine practice now than it once was.

Algorithms

Visual field testing involves estimating the boundaries of an individual's visual field (i.e., where their field of vision stops) as a function of the strength of the visual stimulus (e.g., stimulus size, intensity, and contrast), typically using a statistical algorithm that comes with the hardware. The testing algorithm is generally independent of an individual's results from prior testing sessions. The SITA Standard is a standard algorithm for the Humphrey Field Analyzer; in most cases, this algorithm is used to assess patients initially. More recent algorithms, such as the SITA Fast and SITA Faster, help reduce test duration to minimize patient fatigue.

VARIABILITY AND CHALLENGES IN THE CLINICAL ASSESSMENT OF VISUAL FIELDS

Global indices and reliability indices provide important information for interpreting the results of visual field testing. Multiple factors affect test–retest reliability, and perimetry outcomes can vary as a result of patient-related factors, differences in perimeters and how perimetry is performed, and systems-level factors. Some of these factors can and should be controlled, while others cannot be. All of the factors can impact the quality of the test results, which is important to keep in mind if an individual's results are borderline.

Global Indices

Visual field test results are often summarized using global indices, which provide quantitative measures of overall visual field performance, summarizing information from all the tested locations into a single number. The three most commonly used global indices are mean deviation, pattern standard deviation, and visual field index. Mean deviation represents the average amount of visual field loss, where a lower value indicates greater field loss. Individuals who are more sensitive to stimuli than expected for a normal person of the same age will have positive mean deviation values, whereas those who are less sensitive than expected (i.e., need a brighter stimulus) will have negative mean deviation values, indicating some degree of vision loss (AAO, 2025).

Pattern standard deviation indicates the consistency or asymmetry of the visual field loss across different areas of the field. It is calculated by summing the absolute values of the differences between the normal value for each point and the mean deviation for each point (AAO, 2025). A higher pattern standard deviation value represents a more uneven distribution of field loss, potentially indicating localized damage. Visual field index represents the percentage of the visual field that is still functional, where a lower value represents worse field loss.

Figure 3-6 (h) of the Humphrey visual field printout contains the global indices for that test. The visual field index percent is an alternative measure of overall function, similar to mean deviation in that it reflects the centrally weighted average deviation from the age-matched normal hill of vision but adjusted for average sensitivity. It was developed to characterize diffuse loss caused by cataract and hence emphasizes localized loss more typical of glaucoma (Bengtsson and Heijl, 2008). However, for the severities of visual field loss discussed in this report, visual field index is highly correlated with mean deviation (Artes et al., 2011), and while generalized ("diffuse") loss can be caused by a variety of conditions, removing the effect of generalized loss from nonglaucomatous causes may not always be desirable. The definition of visual field index also includes a change in the way it is calculated at mean deviation of approximately –20 dB, which is the severity of interest for this report. This discontinuity introduces variability when an eye falls just one side or the other of the –20 dB cutoff. Therefore, there are no strong reasons to consider using visual field index rather than mean deviation for SSA disability evaluation.

Reliability Indices

Test reliability in perimetry has traditionally been assessed using three indices: false positives, false negatives, and fixation losses. According to the manufacturer, reliability criteria for past models of the Humphrey Field Analyzer were established as less than 33 percent false-positive error, less than 33 percent false-negative error, and less than 20 percent fixation losses (Newkirk et al., 2006; Ruia and Tripathy, 2023). Today, this guideline exists only for tests not using the SITA family of algorithms.

To illustrate, in the printout of the Humphrey visual field 4-2 SITA Standard Test for a left eye (presented in Figure 3-6), fixation losses measure 3/17, which is less than 20 percent; this is considered a reasonable threshold for reliability based on fixation losses. The false positives measure 6 percent and false negatives 11 percent, which indicates that this test is reliable since both parameters fall below 33 percent. However, binary reliance on these indices is now discouraged, as there is strong evidence that they do not accurately relate to test reliability, as discussed in Chapter 4.

Patient-Related Variability

With respect to patient-related variability, it is important to consider first whether an examinee possesses the mental and physical capacity to participate in the testing, including maintaining a fixed head position and gaze.

Since the validity of the test depends on the person's ability to respond to an illuminated stimulus by pressing a button, factors such as their alertness must be considered. Moreover, a learning curve is associated with perimetric testing, with accuracy of test results improving with repeated testing (Aydin et al., 2015; Heijl and Bengtsson, 1996). When the examinee's mental status is coupled with perimetric experience, the effect on testing validity is notable, with pretest anxiety correlating with test unreliability and likely erroneously indicating the existence of more severe visual field impairment (Chew et al., 2016). Notably, individuals who have undergone ten or more perimetric tests show significantly less anxiety compared with those who have not (Chew et al., 2016).

Other examinee-related factors that can lead to reduced reliability in visual field testing include use of substances such as alcohol, use of medications such as antihistamines and other drugs that may suppress the central nervous system, and the presence of diseases such as diabetes or arthritis (Wild et al., 1988). Fatigue is another factor to be considered. Additionally, individuals with certain ocular conditions (e.g., macular degeneration, diabetic retinopathy) may not be able to fixate, which can be problematic as failure to maintain gaze fixation affects test results. It is therefore important to ensure that the patient understands the test, has the necessary experience to provide an optimal result (e.g., to compensate for the learning curve, to know how to pause the test or when to blink), and has the appropriate modifications to adjust for uncorrected refractive error and other conditions such as dermatochalasis (loose or excess eyelid skin that can result in drooping eyelids that impair the visual field).

Other anatomical factors also influence perimetry results. Chief among these factors is changing eye shape leading to refractive error (such as myopia resulting from elongation of the eye), which requires the appropriate lens correction to ensure that the patient can clearly visualize the stimuli (Johnson, 1996). For example, patients with high myopia may demonstrate less sensitivity, particularly in the cecocentral area (the area around the physiological blind spot), on visual field testing when the 30-2 and 10-2 Humphrey Field Analyzer test patterns are used (Araie et al., 1995). Other investigators have observed specific defects that may be associated with high myopia, such as aberrations around the physiological blind spot; absolute scotomas; and changes in indices such as mean deviation, pattern deviation, and short-term fluctuation (Corallo et al., 1997). Pupil size also may influence perimetric testing results (Lindenmuth et al., 1990). Other notable anatomical factors affecting perimetric reliability include cataracts (Lam et al., 1991), corneal lesions, face shape (Sadegh Mousavi et al., 2024), and dermatochalasis (Kosmin et al., 1997). These anatomical as well as nonanatomical factors have been demonstrated to significantly impact the reliability of perimetric testing (Higginbotham et al., 2003).

Given the variance between individual patient responses during perimetric testing and the difficulty of interpreting nonstereotypic field patterns, it is essential to confirm any detected visual field defects. Repeat visual field tests, using the same program, are needed to confirm visual field loss. Repeat testing is also recommended for examinees who are perimetrically naïve because of the learning curve with most visual field testing, as discussed above (Aydin et al., 2015; Heijl and Bengtsson, 1996). Individuals new to perimetry often need several sessions to achieve reliable outcomes.

Variability in the Assessor, Instrument, and Environment

Perimetry results can vary depending on choices made by practitioners, including the type of perimeter used. For example, earlier versions of the Octopus perimeter presented stimuli following a click sound, which alerted the patient that a stimulus was being projected. Additionally, the order in which the left and right eyes are tested (Searle et al., 1991), the position of the lens holder (Donahue, 1998), and the size of the stimulus (Wall et al., 1997) can each introduce variability and affect test validity.

Some investigators have suggested using different stimulus sizes, instead of the current standard of size III, in testing algorithms. Larger stimuli are easier to detect, increasing the sensitivities, and possibly reducing test–retest variability (Wall et al., 1997). Other investigators have suggested that smaller stimuli may improve the signal-to-noise ratio (Rountree et al., 2018), although those studies have so far focused on detecting early defects rather than discriminating between levels of more severe loss as required for SSA disability assessment. This again emphasizes that the full testing conditions, including the stimulus size and testing algorithm, need to be considered when deciding whether a test is suitable for assessment of disability, rather than only considering the perimeter used.

Supervision of individuals during testing has been demonstrated to ensure that they remain awake and are well positioned during the test and that unnecessary distraction is minimized (Johnson, 1996). Thus, it is generally considered important that the technician remain in the room with the examinee to ensure optimal conditions. However, if a professional staff member cannot be present, alternative strategies, such as the use of a training video before the test starts, may yield similar results (Maheshwari et al., 2023).

Challenges and Opportunities in Systems-Level Factors

Visual field testing using traditional perimeters, such as the Humphrey Field Analyzer (static automated threshold perimeter) and the Octopus (combined static automated threshold and semiautomated kinetic perimeter), requires oversight by a vision specialist, such as an optometrist or ophthalmologist. Vision screening and care can be more difficult for some groups of people to access than others. For example, people living in rural communities and urban communities of color have individuals with more severe retinopathy and less access to eye care relative to other groups (Hale et al., 2010; Sommer et al., 1991). Fewer eye clinics accept Medicaid compared with private insurance, many clinics have appointments booked out several months, and out-of-pocket costs can be high. Lack of transportation can also be an issue. As the U.S. population ages, one can expect higher patient volumes in the next few decades without an increase in vision specialists (Hughes et al., 2022; Mehrotra and Uscher-Pines, 2022; NASEM, 2016; Sinsky et al., 2021).

One way to expand access to vision testing is through teleophthalmology. Teleophthalmology can provide evidence-based diabetic eye screening for people with diabetes by, for example, making it possible to conduct the testing in a primary care setting and send results electronically to eye specialists, who can then provide a diabetic retinopathy report and a clinical evaluation and treatment plan (Horton et al., 2020; Liu et al., 2019). This type of testing is fast and inexpensive. Other potential settings for vision screening and care include health clinics and federally qualified health centers. The latter are primary care–based, safety-net community clinics that are located throughout the United States and provide medical care regardless of insurance type or insurance status. Finally, new technologies in visual field testing that do not require expensive equipment show promise for increasing access to visual field testing. The next section introduces some of these new technologies.

RECENT CHANGES IN PRACTICE

This section reviews emerging perimetric technologies and advances in perimetric testing algorithms, as well as the implications of these advances for SSA's disability evaluation.

Emerging Technologies

Several new perimetric technologies have been developed in recent years.

Virtual Reality Headsets

Virtual reality (VR) headsets can be used to present stimuli to individual eyes. The viewing distance is small, but with a suitably high screen resolution the stimulus can be made indistinguishable to the observer from a stimulus in a traditional bowl perimeter. Some VR systems have built-in eye tracking, which can provide an accurate measure of fixation stability and hence ensure the reliability of test results. Certain individuals may find the weight of the headset uncomfortable, but others prefer it to a traditional perimeter because their head does not have to remain in a fixed position leaning forward onto a chin rest, a particular benefit for people with neck or back pain. The headset typically blocks out extraneous light, so the testing no longer needs be performed in a darkened room, which greatly increases flexibility for the location of the testing. Thus, the testing may be performed in waiting rooms or in settings outside of eye clinics, although it should be noted that audible distractions in those settings could themselves impact test reliability.

At the time this report was being prepared, the Food and Drug Administration (FDA) had approved three VR devices for perimetry, and more portable devices are likely to receive FDA approval in the next 5 years. A growing literature over the last decade supports the use of these new devices as valid and reliable alternatives to traditional perimetry. Chapter 4 offers insight into how those studies can be evaluated.

imo Head-Mounted Perimeter and Topcon Tempo Perimeter

The imo head-mounted automated perimeter (Figure 3-9) is an emerging technology that provides a more portable option relative to traditional perimeters such as the Humphrey Field Analyzer and Octopus (Ishibashi et al., 2022; Matsumoto et al., 2016). The device consists of a "head-mounted perimeter unit, a separate response button and a tablet which is controlled by the operator" (Wu et al., 2022). This device measures within 35 degrees of the center of the visual field (Matsumoto et al., 2016). An alternative desk-based version of the hardware has also been released as the Topcon Tempo perimeter, with the same testing algorithms. Testing with the imo can be performed as either a monocular test (since there are two testing systems, one for each eye) or a binocular random single-eye test. The imo also includes a

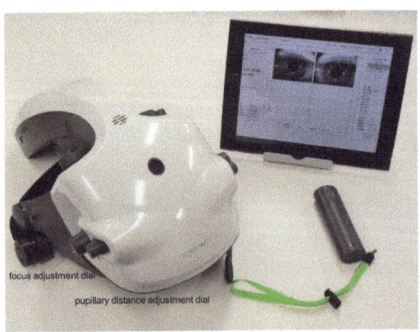 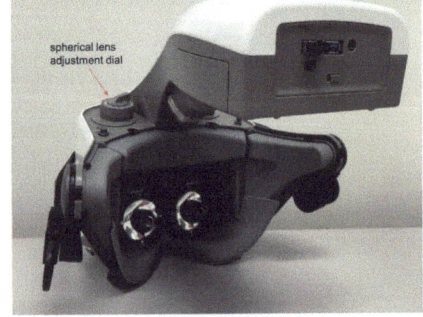

FIGURE 3-9 imo head-mounted automated perimeter.
SOURCE: Matsumoto et al. (2016). CC0 1.0.

unique testing strategy—the "24 plus"—which includes 78 points, 54 within the 24-2 pattern and an additional 24 in the central 10-degree visual field. A comparison of the imo device and the Humphrey Field Analyzer in patients with glaucoma found no significant difference in mean deviation results; however, testing time was shorter for the imo than for the Humphrey Field Analyzer (Kimura et al., 2019). A new algorithm, described in the next section, was developed for use with the imo device.

iCare Compass

The iCare Compass is a static automated threshold perimeter combined with an active retinal tracker and a scanning ophthalmoscope. This design enables simultaneous retinal imaging during the visual field test, and hence more accurate comparison of structural and functional measurements. For the purposes of SSA disability evaluation, the relevant difference from the above instruments is that retinal tracking adjusts for, and so reduces, fixation losses. Mean deviation measurements tend to correlate well between the Compass and the Humprey Field Analyzer, including at the severities of interest for SSA assessment (Liu et al., 2021; Montesano et al., 2019).

Tablet and Desktop Computer–Based Testing

An alternative approach to head-mounted devices is to perform the testing on a tablet or desktop computer. These devices are widely available and already owned by a large and ever-increasing proportion of individuals, making home testing more feasible with these devices than with VR headsets, which have higher cost and far lower ownership rates. Use of such devices also expands testing availability beyond clinics with bowl perimeters.

The primary advantage of using tablets and desktop computers for visual field testing is increased accessibility. However, use of these devices has disadvantages as well. The main disadvantage is the lack of standardization of test conditions. Background light levels are not controlled; viewing distances (and hence angles) may not be consistent or accurate; the screen may not always be angled perpendicular to the viewing angle; and stimulus brightness can vary both temporally (because of hardware degradation over time) and spatially (because of dirt on the screen). A further consideration is that binocular instead of monocular viewing is often used, whether by design or as a result of test subjects not following the detailed directions. This makes it impossible to use the standard catch trial method for assessing fixation losses, since stimuli cannot be presented within the physiological blind spot; therefore, it becomes necessary to employ automated eye tracking, which is not possible with many of the commercial devices present in people's homes. In addition, screen sizes may be too small to measure the necessary spatial extent of the visual field. Although this issue can be ameliorated by having the test subject fixate on one side or one corner of the screen, doing so comes at the cost of increased eye movement (loss of fixation) because the examinee knows in advance the region of the visual field in which the stimulus will appear. Another caveat is that some of these devices can present only a limited range of stimulus contrasts because of hardware limitations.

Tablets and desktop computers offer other advantages over bowl perimeters. They are much cheaper and far more portable and can be more flexible with regard to testing conditions and settings. They allow use of stimulus types other than a static white-on-white circle—for example, spatially varying flickering stimuli, such as a Gabor patch (see Figure 3-10), that cannot be presented using a projection-based bowl perimeter. This feature may be particularly useful for pediatric testing since more engaging stimuli can be used. If designed and implemented well and with adequate built-in instructions, tablets and desktop computers can reduce or even eliminate the need for testing to be performed by a trained technician without precluding reliability. Given the caveats concerning reduced standardization of testing conditions, it is essential to ensure that they have equivalent reliability for assessing visual disability when used in the intended setting.

Short-Wavelength Automated Perimetry

An additional testing mode available on the Humphrey Field Analyzer is short-wavelength automated perimetry (SWAP). This test isolates cells

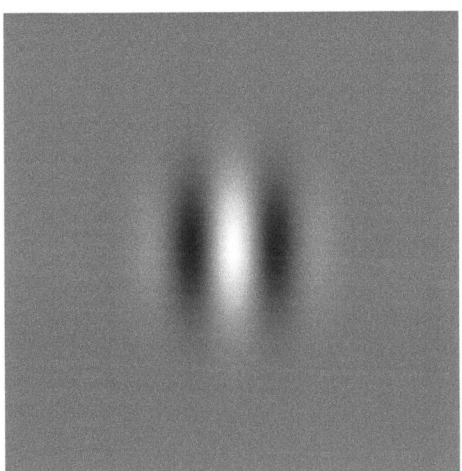

FIGURE 3-10 Example of a Gabor patch.
SOURCE: Tsushima et al. (2020). CC BY 4.0.

sensitive to short wavelengths by projecting a narrow band of blue-light stimulus on a bowl illuminated with a yellow light. The size of the target is equivalent to a Goldmann size V. The background reduces the sensitivities of the green and red cones, isolating the short wavelength–sensitive blue cones and their associated small, bistratified retinal ganglion cells. SWAP is considered to be more sensitive to early glaucoma than standard perimetry. A study designed to assess the role and diagnostic capability of optical coherence tomography and SWAP in distinguishing among normal eyes, glaucoma suspects, and diagnosed glaucomatous eyes found both to be effective tools for this purpose (Zaky et al., 2016). However, SWAP showed superior ability to detect glaucomatous changes in the glaucoma suspect group.

Despite the promise of SWAP to detect glaucomatous field loss prior to structural changes in the optic nerve, its clinical use has limitations. Greater variability in testing has been noted with SWAP compared with static automated threshold perimetry (Blumenthal et al., 2000). Moreover, limitations of previous comparative studies of SWAP and static automated threshold perimetry include the lack of a standardized age-corrected normal database for SWAP and the absence of statistically and clinically robust criteria for defining abnormality or progressive loss for SWAP. These limitations, among others, have hindered understanding of SWAP's effectiveness in detecting progressive loss in glaucoma and have made it challenging to determine whether SWAP offers any significant advantages over white-on-white perimetry, beyond SWAP's core function of detecting field loss earlier (Wild, 2001).

Given the above factors, as well as the fact that SWAP is designed to detect early defects in the visual field, it does not appear to be suitable for SSA's use in determining disability benefits. However, studies conducted on SWAP over the last two decades have yielded lessons about the elements of clinical studies that are needed to assess the viability of new perimetric devices on the horizon. As described in Chapter 4, the number of studies is not as critical as their quality in ensuring that any given test provides the information needed to assess the ability of visually impaired individuals to function.

Advances in Testing Algorithms

As noted previously, the Humphrey Field Analyzer is the most commonly used perimeter in clinical practice in the United States. In most cases in current practice, the Humphrey SITA Standard Threshold Test is used for initial patient assessment. SITA shortens the number of stimuli posed to the patient relative to the original Full Threshold strategy, which is almost never used today, and quickly learns which additional points should be tested based on previous responses. SITA Fast was introduced to further shorten testing time. Both SITA Standard and SITA Fast reduce testing time and are similarly sensitive for detecting moderate and severe glaucoma (Budenz et al., 2002). More recently, even faster algorithms have been developed to shorten the identification of defects without jeopardizing the reliability of the test (Budenz et al., 2002; Wu et al., 2022).

To reduce the variability that exists in perimetric testing when patients are fatigued because of the test's long duration, investigators developed SITA Faster, a modified version of the SITA Fast perimetric testing strategy designed to reduce the number of stimulus presentations while maintaining accuracy in visual field testing. It incorporates several modifications to enhance efficiency and potentially increase the frequency of perimetric testing, which is important for earlier detection of progression in conditions such as glaucoma. The aim of developing this software was to provide a shorter testing duration without compromising the effectiveness of glaucoma detection compared with SITA Fast and SITA Standard. The development of SITA Faster involved simulations and clinical testing, and it has been evaluated in a multicenter clinical study (Heijl et al., 2019). That study found that the mean test times for SITA Faster were significantly shorter than for SITA Fast and SITA Standard, and the results for mean deviation were similar among all three tests at all severities. The visual field index did not differ between SITA Fast and SITA Faster, but the values were found to be lower with SITA Standard than with both SITA Fast and SITA Faster. Additionally, there was a slightly higher number of significantly damaged test points with SITA Standard than with SITA Fast and SITA Faster. All three tests exhibited similar test–retest variability across the entire range of threshold values in all groups. Overall, SITA Faster demonstrated considerable time savings while providing results comparable to those obtained with SITA Fast (Heijl et al., 2019). However, SITA Faster would not be acceptable to SSA currently because it does not automatically perform the false-negative catch trials that SSA prefers, although this function can be activated by the operator.

Another new algorithm, the Ambient Interactive Zippy Estimation by Sequential Testing (AIZE) algorithm, was developed for use with the imo head-mounted perimeter. The AIZE algorithm shortens testing time and has been demonstrated to have equivalent mean deviation as reported by the Humphrey Field Analyzer 24-2 testing strategies across the full range of damage severities (Nishida et al., 2023).

Implications for Disability Evaluation

Testing algorithms are not mentioned in SSA's Listing of Impairments for Special Senses and Speech (SSA, n.d.-a, -b), but the choice of algorithm is potentially important, as performance is algorithm specific. As visual field loss worsens, variability in performance increases. For individuals who are sufficiently impaired to be categorized as disabled, variability will be greater. Given the learning curve, conducting multiple tests might improve the accuracy of the results. It is unclear how many visual field tests might be required to achieve optimum accuracy, but a minimum of two tests could be expected to improve the accuracy of results. Physician notes are also important to consider.

With respect to testing patterns, SSA's listing criteria for assessing mean deviation require a Humphrey Field Analyzer 30-2 test result. The committee points out that the 30-2 testing pattern is used less often now in routine practice than it used to be, and the 30-2 and 24-2 patterns are functionally equivalent in most cases. Nevertheless, the SITA 30-2 algorithm can be helpful in specialized clinical settings, such neuro-ophthalmology, and certain research settings. Kinetic perimetry is also not routinely used and not needed except for special circumstances, such as for SSA's calculation of visual field efficiency, as well as special use cases detailed in Chapter 5.

SUMMARY AND CONCLUSIONS

Perimetry, also known as visual field testing, is an essential diagnostic tool for assessing various ophthalmic conditions, including glaucoma, optic neuropathies, and disorders affecting the retina and visual pathways. Perimetry techniques consist of a combination of hardware, stimuli, testing patterns, and algorithms. The Humphrey Field Analyzer (static automated threshold perimeter) is the most widely used perimeter in the United States, with the Octopus perimeter (combined static automated threshold and semiautomated kinetic perimeter) also commonly being used, particularly in Europe. The Humphrey Field Analyzer employs specialized algorithms such as SITA Standard and SITA Fast, with testing patterns such as 30-2, 24-2, and 10-2, allowing targeted assessment of the central visual field, as well as more peripheral areas. Stimulus presentation varies across perimetry systems. While optical projection is standard, some devices now use LCD-based stimuli for consistent brightness and contrast.

SAP using white-on-white stimuli measures the sensitivity of an individual's visual field at specific test locations and has the capability to compare the findings with a database of previously tested patients with normal vision. Specific programs can be used to tailor the visual field test to focus on distinct areas of a patient's concentrated visual field loss. Manual or semiautomated kinetic perimetry may also be used by eye care providers to assess the visual field. However, because semiautomated kinetic perimetry does not require trained personnel to conduct and because it provides the capability to standardize testing conditions, it is more commonly used.

Recent changes in practice include newer algorithms, such as SITA Fast and SITA Faster for the Humphrey Field Analyzer, that shorten the number of stimuli posed to the patient and can quickly learn which additional points should be tested based on previous responses. Shorter testing times decrease reliability, although not significantly. Generally, patients who may be suspected of conditions such as glaucoma may initially undergo a 24-2 test using the Humphrey Field Analyzer. Other potential testing protocols include the Humphrey Field Analyzer SITA 10-2 if loss is suspected close to central fixation and the patient is suspected of demonstrating advanced field loss; the Humphrey Field Analyzer SITA 30-2, which covers a greater expanse of the visual field, can be used if more peripheral loss is expected.

Testing algorithms are not mentioned in the SSA listings, but they are important, as performance is algorithm specific. As the visual field loss worsens, variability in performance increases. For individuals who are sufficiently impaired to be categorized as disabled, variability will be greater. Given the learning curve, conducting multiple tests might improve the accuracy of the results. It is unclear how many visual field tests might be required to achieve optimum accuracy, but conducting a minimum of two tests could be expected to improve the accuracy of results, particularly in patients naïve to visual field tests.

With respect to testing patterns, SSA's listing criteria for assessing mean deviation require a Humphrey Field Analyzer 30-2 test result. The committee points out that the 30-2 testing pattern is used less often now than it once was, and the 30-2 and 24-2 patterns are functionally equivalent in many instances. Nevertheless, the SITA 30-2 algorithm can be helpful in specialized clinical settings, such neuro-ophthalmology and certain research settings. Kinetic perimetry is also not routinely used and not needed except for special circumstances such as for SSA's calculation of visual field efficiency.

Based on its review of the literature, the committee reached the following conclusions:

Conclusion 3.1: Measurement of visual field impairment involves components beyond the hardware or visual perimetry device, including stimuli, testing patterns, and algorithms. All components are important to consider when evaluating the validity of visual field assessment.

Conclusion 3.2: Because variability in the results of visual field assessment increases as the severity of visual field impairment increases, and given the learning curve in visual field testing, more than one visual field test may be needed to characterize an individual's visual field impairment accurately.

Conclusion 3.3: The Social Security Administration's listing criteria for assessing mean deviation require a Humphrey Field Analyzer 30-2 test result, but this testing pattern is used less often now in routine practice. In many instances, however, the 24-2 testing pattern is functionally equivalent to the 30-2 testing pattern and may be sufficient for assessing mean deviation.

Perimetry outcomes can vary because of patient-related factors, differences in perimeters and how perimetry is performed, and systems-level factors. Patient-level factors include whether a patient possesses the mental and physical capacity to participate in the testing, the patient's previous experience with perimetric testing, their use of alcohol and medications that may suppress the central nervous system, the presence of diseases such as diabetes or arthritis, fatigue, and ocular conditions that may affect their ability to fixate. Perimetry results also can vary depending on choices practitioners make, including the type of perimeter used, the order in which the left and right eyes are tested, and whether patients are supervised and well positioned during the testing. In terms of systems-level factors, visual field testing using traditional perimeters, such as the Humphrey Field Analyzer (static automated) and Octopus (combined static automated threshold and semiautomated kinetic), requires oversight by experienced technicians, creating challenges for individuals with limited access to appropriately trained eye care providers. With an aging population and insufficient numbers of eye care providers projected in the future, teleophthalmology offers a solution by enabling remote diabetic eye screenings and evaluations. Expanding vision care to settings such as primary care, health clinics, and federally qualified health centers could improve access. Emerging, cost-effective technologies, such as virtual reality headsets and tablet- and desktop-based systems, also show promise for improving accessibility. With proper design and implementation, these tools could significantly expand access to visual field testing while maintaining reliability.

Based on its review of the literature, the committee reached the following conclusion:

Conclusion 3.4: Visual field testing with traditional perimeters such as the Humphrey Field Analyzer and Octopus requires oversight by experienced technicians who may be in limited supply, creating challenges for some populations with limited access to care. Emerging cost-effective technologies, such as virtual reality headsets and tablet- and desktop-based systems, show promise for improving accessibility. With proper design and implementation, these tools may significantly expand access to visual field testing while maintaining reliability and validity, assuming studies demonstrate the ability to provide accurate, reproducible results even in an unsupervised setting and their suitability for determining SSA disability in the target population.

REFERENCES

AAO (American Academy of Ophthalmology). 2020. *Primary open-angle glaucoma preferred practice pattern.* https://www.aaojournal.org/action/showPdf?pii=S0161-6420%2820%2931024-1 (accessed February 25, 2025).

AAO. 2025. *Standard automated perimetry.* EyeWiki. https://eyewiki.org/Standard_Automated_Perimetry (accessed February 24, 2025).

AOA (American Optometric Association). 2024. *Care of the patient with primary open-angle glaucoma,* 1st ed. https://www.aoa.org/a/19461 (accessed March 24, 2025).

Araie, M., M. Arai, N. Koseki, and Y. Suzuki. 1995. Influence of myopic refraction on visual field defects in normal tension and primary open angle glaucoma. *Japanese Journal of Ophthalmology* 39(1):60–64.

Artes, P. H., N. O'Leary, D. M. Hutchison, L. Heckler, G. P. Sharpe, M. T. Nicolela, and B. C. Chauhan. 2011. Properties of the statpac visual field index. *Investigative Ophthalmology & Visual Science* 52(7):4030–4038.

Aydin, A., İ. Koçak, U. Aykan, G. Can, M. Sabahyildizi, and D. Ersanli. 2015. The influence of the learning effect on automated perimetry in a Turkish population. *Journal Francais d'Ophtalmologie* 38(7):628–632.

Bengtsson, B., and A. Heijl. 2008. A visual field index for calculation of glaucoma rate of progression. *American Journal of Ophthalmology* 145(2):343–353.

Blumenthal, E. Z., P. A. Sample, L. Zangwill, A. C. Lee, Y. Kono, and R. N. Weinreb. 2000. Comparison of long-term variability for standard and short-wavelength automated perimetry in stable glaucoma patients. *American Journal of Ophthalmology* 129(3):309–313.

Budenz, D. L., P. Rhee, W. J. Feuer, J. McSoley, C. A. Johnson, and D. R. Anderson. 2002. Sensitivity and specificity of the Swedish interactive threshold algorithm for glaucomatous visual field defects. *Ophthalmology* 109(6):1052–1058.

Chew, S. S., N. M. Kerr, A. B. Wong, J. P. Craig, C.-Y. Chou, and H. V. Danesh-Meyer. 2016. Anxiety in visual field testing. *British Journal of Ophthalmology* 100(8):1128–1133.

Corallo, G., P. Capris, and M. Zingirian. 1997. Perimetric findings in subjects with elevated myopia and glaucoma. *Acta Ophthalmologica Scandinavica* 75(S224):30–31.

Damato, B. E. 1985. Oculokinetic perimetry: A simple visual field test for use in the community. *The British Journal of Ophthalmology* 69(12):927–931.

Donahue, S. P. 1998. Lens holder artifact simulating glaucomatous defect in automated perimetry. *Archives of Ophthalmology* 116(12):1681–1683.

Hale, N. L., K. J. Bennett, and J. C. Probst. 2010. Diabetes care and outcomes: Disparities across rural America. *Journal of Community Health* 35(4):365–374.

Heijl, A., and B. Bengtsson. 1996. The effect of perimetric experience in patients with glaucoma. *Archives of Ophthalmology* 114(1):19–22.

Heijl, A., V. M. Patella, and B. Bengtsson. 2021. *The field analyzer primer: Excellent perimetry*, 5th ed. Carl Zeiss Meditec, Inc.

Heijl, A., V. M. Patella, L. X. Chong, A. Iwase, C. K. Leung, A. Tuulonen, G. C. Lee, T. Callan, and B. Bengtsson. 2019. A New SITA perimetric threshold testing algorithm: Construction and a multicenter clinical study. *American Journal of Ophthalmology* 198:154–165.

Henley, C. 2021. *Foundations of neuroscience*, open edition. Michigan State University. https://openbooks.lib.msu.edu/neuroscience/chapter/vision-the-retina/

Higginbotham, E. J., N. Ellish, and R. Kalsi. 2003. The variability of perimetry: Reassessing an important clinical tool. In *Glaucoma in the new millennium: Proceedings of the 50th annual symposium on glaucoma, New Orleans, LA, USA, April 6-8, 2001, Organized by the New Orleans Academy of Ophthalmology*. Monroe, NY: Kugler Publications.

Horton, M. B., C. J. Brady, J. Cavallerano, M. Abramoff, G. Barker, M. F. Chiang, C. H. Crockett, S. Garg, P. Karth, Y. Liu, C. D. Newman, S. Rathi, V. Sheth, P. Silva, K. Stebbins, and I. Zimmer-Galler. 2020. Practice guidelines for ocular telehealth—Diabetic retinopathy, 3rd ed. *Telemedicine and e-Health* 26(4):495–543.

Hughes, H. K., B. W. Hasselfeld, and J. A. Greene. 2022. Health care access on the line—audio-only visits and digitally inclusive care. *New England Journal of Medicine* 387(20):1823–1826.

Ishibashi, T., C. Matsumoto, H. Nomoto, F. Tanabe, I. Narita, M. Ishibashi, S. Okuyama, T. Kayazawa, S. Kimura, K. Yamanaka, and S. Kusaka. 2022. Measurement of fixational eye movements with the head-mounted perimeter imo. *Translational Vision Science & Technology* 11(8):26. https://doi.org/10.1167/tvst.11.8.26

Johnson, C. A. 1996. Standardizing the measurement of visual fields for clinical research: Guidelines from the eye care technology forum. *Ophthalmology* 103(1):186–189.

Kimura, T., C. Matsumoto, and H. Nomoto. 2019. Comparison of head-mounted perimeter (imo®) and Humphrey Field Analyzer. *Clinical Ophthalmology* 13:501.

Kolb, H. 1995. Simple anatomy of the retina. In H. Kolb, R. Nelson, E. Fernandez, and B. Jones (Eds.), *Webvision: The organization of the retina and visual system*. University of Utah Health Sciences Center. https://webvision.med.utah.edu/book/part-i-foundations/simple-anatomy-of-the-retina/ (accessed April 1, 2025).

Kosmin, A. S., P. K. Wishart, and M. K. Birch. 1997. Apparent glaucomatous visual field defects caused by dermatochalasis. *Eye* 11(5):682–686.

Lam, B. L., W. L. Alward, and H. E. Kolder. 1991. Effect of cataract on automated perimetry. *Ophthalmology* 98(7):1066–1070.

Lindenmuth, K. A., G. L. Skuta, R. Rabbani, D. C. Musch, and T. J. Bergstrom. 1990. Effects of pupillary dilation on automated perimetry in normal patients. *Ophthalmology* 97(3):367–370.

Liu, P., B. N. Nguyen, A. Turpin, and A. M. McKendrick. 2021. Increased depth, reduced extent, and sharpened edges of visual field defects measured by compass fundus perimeter compared to Humphrey field analyzer. *Translational Vision Science & Technology* 10(12):33.

Liu, Y., A. Torres Diaz, and R. Benkert. 2019. Scaling up teleophthalmology for diabetic eye screening: Opportunities for widespread implementation in the USA. *Current Diabetes Reports* 19:74.

Maheshwari, D., A. Nair, T. D. Tara, N. Pawar, R. Ramakrishnan, D. R. G. Selvi, and M. S. Uduman. 2023. Comparison of the effect of audiovisual and verbal instructions on patient performance while performing automated Humphrey Visual Field testing. *Indian Journal of Ophthalmology* 71(2):569–574.

Matsumoto, C., S. Yamao, H. Nomoto, S. Takada, S. Okuyama, S. Kimura, K. Yamanaka, M. Aihara, and Y. Shimomura. 2016. Visual field testing with head-mounted perimeter 'imo'. *PLoS One* 11(8):e0161974.

Mehrotra, A., and L. Uscher-Pines. 2022. Informing the debate about telemedicine reimbursement—what do we need to know? *New England Journal of Medicine* 387(20):1821–1823.

Montesano, G., S. R. Bryan, D. P. Crabb, P. Fogagnolo, F. Oddone, A. M. McKendrick, A. Turpin, P. Lanzetta, A. Perdicchi, C. A. Johnson, D. F. Garway-Heath, P. Brusini, and L. M. Rossetti. 2019. A comparison between the compass fundus perimeter and the Humphrey field analyzer. *Ophthalmology* 126(2):242–251.

Murray, I. C., Fleck, B. W., Brash, H. M., Macrae, M. E., Tan, L. L., & Minns, R. A. (2009). Feasibility of saccadic vector optokinetic perimetry: A method of automated static perimetry for children using eye tracking. *Ophthalmology*, 116(10):2017–2026.

NASEM (National Academies of Sciences, Engineering, and Medicine). 2016. *Making eye health a population health imperative: Vision for tomorrow*. Washington, DC: The National Academies Press.

Newkirk, M. R., S. K. Gardiner, S. Demirel, and C. A. Johnson. 2006. Assessment of false positives with the Humphrey Field Analyzer II perimeter with the SITA algorithm. *Investigative Ophthalmology & Visual Science* 47(10):4632–4637.

Nieto, M. P. 2015. *A simplified schema of the human visual pathway*. https://commons.wikimedia.org/wiki/User:Perellonieto#/media/File:Human_visual_pathway.svg

Nishida, T., R. N. Weinreb, J. Arias, C. Vasile, and S. Moghimi. 2023. Comparison of the TEMPO binocular perimeter and Humphrey Field Analyzer. *Scientific Reports* 13:21189.

Racette, L., M. Fischer, H. Bebie, G. Hollo, C. A. Johnson, and C. Matsumoto. 2019. *Visual field digest: A guide to perimetry and the Octopus perimeter, 8th ed.* https://haag-streit.com/2%20Products/Speciality%20diagnostics/Perimetry/Category%20assets/Books/HS_perimetry_br_xxx_visual_field_digest_8th_en.pdf (accessed February 3, 2025).

Rountree, L., P. J. Mulholland, R. S. Anderson, D. F. Garway-Heath, J. E. Morgan, and T. Redmond. 2018. Optimising the glaucoma signal/noise ratio by mapping changes in spatial summation with area-modulated perimetric stimuli. *Scientific Reports*:8(1):2172.

Ruia, S., and K. Tripathy. 2023. *Humphrey visual field*. StatPearls [Internet]. https://www.ncbi.nlm.nih.gov/books/NBK585112/ (accessed February 11, 2025).

Sadegh Mousavi, S., S. Jamali Dogahe, L. J. Lyons, and C. L. Khanna. 2024. Head turn during visual field testing to minimize the influence of prominent facial anatomy. *Journal of Neuro-Ophthalmology* 44(2):253–258.

Schiefer, U., J. Pätzold, and F. Dannheim. 2005. Conventional perimetry I: Introduction—basics. *Ophthalmologe* 102(6):627–644.

Searle, A. E., J. M. Wild, D. E. Shaw, and E. C. O'Neill. 1991. Time-related variation in normal automated static perimetry. *Ophthalmology* 98(5):701–707.

Sikorski, B. L., and A. Laudencka. 2020. Comparison of advanced threshold and SITA fast perimetric strategies. *Journal of Ophthalmology* 2020:7139649.

Sinsky, C. A., J. T. Jerzak, and K. D. Hopkins. 2021. Telemedicine and team-based care: The perils and the promise. *Mayo Clinic Proceedings* 96(2):429–437.

Sommer, A., J. M. Tielsch, J. Katz, H. A. Quigley, J. D. Gottsch, J. Javitt, J. F. Martone, R. M. Royall, K. A. Witt, and S. Ezrine. 1991. Racial differences in the cause-specific prevalence of blindness in east Baltimore. *New England Journal of Medicine* 325(20):1412–1417.

SSA (U.S. Social Security Administration). n.d.-a. Disability evaluation under social security: *Social Security—2.00 special senses and speech—Adult*. https://www.ssa.gov/disability/professionals/bluebook/2.00-SpecialSensesandSpeech-Adult.htm (accessed February 3, 2025).

SSA. n.d.-b. *Disability evaluation under Social Security—102.00 special senses and speech—Childhood*. https://www.ssa.gov/disability/professionals/bluebook/102.00-SpecialSensesandSpeech-Childhood.htm (accessed February 3, 2025).

Talib, M., G. Dagnelie, and C. J. F. Boon. 2018. Recording and analysis of Goldmann kinetic visual fields. *Methods in Molecular Biology* 1715:327–338.

Traquair, H. M. 1947. *An introduction to clinical perimetry*, 6th ed. London: Henry Kimpton Press.

Tsushima, Y., Y. Sawahata, and K. Komine. 2020. Task-dependent fMRI decoder with the power to extend Gabor patch results to natural images. *Scientific Reports* 10(1):1382. https://doi.org/10.1038/s41598-020-58241-x

Wall, M., K. E. Kutzko, and B. C. Chauhan. 1997. Variability in patients with glaucomatous visual field damage is reduced using size V stimuli. *Investigative Ophthalmology & Visual Science* 38(2):426–435.

Weber, J., and J. Caprioli. 2000. *Atlas of computerized perimetry*. Saunders.

Wild, J., T. Betts, K. Ross, and C. Kenwood. 1988. Influence of antihistamines on central visual field assessment. *Perimetry Update* 1989:439–445.

Wild, J. M. 2001. Short wavelength automated perimetry. *Acta Ophthalmologica Scandinavica* 79(6):546–559.

Wong, S. H., and G. T. Plant. 2015. How to interpret visual fields. *Practical Neurology* 15(5):374–381. https://doi.org/10.1136/practneurol-2015-001155

Wu, Y., M. Szymanska, Y. Hu, M. I. Fazal, N. Jiang, A. K. Yetisen, and M. F. Cordeiro. 2022. Measures of disease activity in glaucoma. *Biosensors and Bioelectronics* 196:113700.

Zaky, A. G., A. T. Yassin, and S. H. El Sayid. 2016. Short wave–automated perimetry (SWAP) versus optical coherence tomography in early detection of glaucoma. *Clinical Ophthalmology* 19(10):1819–1824.

4

Evaluating New Perimetry Techniques

As noted previously, perimetry techniques consist of hardware, stimuli, testing patterns, and algorithms in combination; one of the components cannot be assessed without the others being specified. In evaluating a perimetry technique, the key consideration is not just how measurements are obtained but whether the technique demonstrates acceptable performance for the relevant task. This chapter first presents considerations for the design of studies for assessing the accuracy of diagnostic tests, then provides an in-depth discussion of performance considerations for assessing new perimetry techniques. The chapter concludes with a discussion of the question from the committee's statement of task on the quantity and characteristics of validation studies needed to find a perimeter acceptable.

DESIGN OF STUDIES FOR ASSESSING DIAGNOSTIC TEST ACCURACY[1]

Determining whether an individual meets the Social Security Administration's (SSA's) criteria for disability benefit eligibility is fundamentally a classification task, aligning with recognized principles for the design and evaluation of studies of diagnostic tests, as set forth in the *Cochrane Handbook for Systematic Reviews of Diagnostic Test Accuracy* (Deeks et al., 2023). The design of such a study fundamentally involves recruiting as participants a single group of individuals, all of whom are *suspected* of

---

[1] The committee relied on the *Cochrane Handbook for Systematic Reviews of Diagnostic Test Accuracy* (Deeks et al., 2023) for much of the content of this section.

having the condition of interest. It is essential for this group to be representative of and drawn from the target population or intended-use population in the relevant setting (e.g., primary care, specialty care). Otherwise, spectrum bias can occur—that is, the study participants may not adequately represent the full range ("spectrum") of patients one would expect to see in the intended setting. Thus, the study population could overrepresent some groups (e.g., those with more severe forms of the condition of interest) or underrepresent others (e.g., those whose condition is in an early stage or is of a milder form). Spectrum bias can then lead to either overestimation or underestimation of the real-world performance of the diagnostic test whose accuracy is being assessed.

In such a study, the test being assessed—referred to as the index test—is administered to each of the study participants. This index test may involve a new device (e.g., a tablet-based device or one that employs a virtual reality headset), or the use of a new testing algorithm with an existing device, or a combination of a new device and a new algorithm or other component(s) of a perimetry technique. Shortly thereafter, participants undergo a different test termed the reference standard. The reference standard is usually the best clinical method available for determining whether patients have the target condition (hence it is sometimes called the "gold standard," although it is seldom 100 percent accurate, particularly in the case of visual field testing). The reference standard used most frequently in visual field testing is the perimetry technique most commonly used in clinical practice today—a 24-2 testing pattern on the Humphrey Field Analyzer using a Goldmann size III (0.43-degree diameter) stimulus and the Swedish Interactive Threshold Algorithm (SITA)—although other reference standards have also been used (Table 4-1).

Once participants have undergone both the index test and the reference standard, the two sets of results are compared for each participant. Those comparisons are then aggregated to form an estimate of the accuracy (e.g., sensitivity and/or specificity) of the index test in the intended setting and for the target population. This comparison is not, by itself, sufficient evidence to accept a new diagnostic test; other factors such as reproducibility must also be considered (see below). In fact, test–retest variability (i.e., reproducibility) may affect the amount of intertest variability found in an individual study. To examine this, researchers occasionally examine test–retest variability for both the index test and the reference standard. More commonly, however, they will simply compare against values for test–retest variability found in the literature.

Diagnostic test accuracy studies are inherently cross-sectional, aiming to assess a test's performance in identifying patients with the condition of interest at the time the test was conducted. The fully paired study design described above employs a single set of inclusion and exclusion criteria for study participants that define the target population from which the group

TABLE 4-1 Reference Standards Used in Perimetry Validation Studies

Citation	Index Test under Evaluation	Reference Standard
Ahmed et al., 2022	Toronto Portable Perimeter (virtual reality [VR] headset using smartphone)	HFA, SITA Standard 24-2, size III stimulus
Balasubramanian et al., 2023 (conference abstract)	LED perimeter	Octopus 900, unknown algorithm, size V stimulus
Bentley et al., 2012	Useful Field of View	HFA, SITA Standard 24-2, size III stimulus; HFA binocular Esterman program (functional test evaluating fitness to drive)
Bradley et al., 2024	Radius Virtual Reality Perimeter	HFA, SITA Standard 24-2, size III stimulus
Chen et al., 2022	LUXIE (head-mounted VR with eye tracking)	HFA, SITA Standard 30-2, size III stimulus
Chen et al., 2024	Perimouse (computer-based, website)	HFA, SITA Standard 24-2, size III stimulus
Chia et al., 2019	Melbourne Rapid Fields (tablet based)	HFA or Octopus 600, SITA or Octopus Standard 24-2, size III stimulus
Chia et al., 2021	Melbourne Rapid Fields (tablet based)	HFA or Octopus 600, SITA or Octopus Standard 24-2, size III stimulus
Crossland et al., 2011	Adapted microperimeter	Modified HFA, matrix mapping algorithm, size III stimulus
Cui et al., 2019	Heidelberg Edge Perimeter	Octopus 900, G-TOP (tendency-oriented perimetry) 30-2, size III stimulus
Heinzman et al., 2022	VR headset	Octopus 900, Zippy Estimation by Sequential Testing (ZEST), size V stimulus
Heinzman et al., 2023	Iowa Head-Mounted Display Open-Source Perimeter	Octopus 900, ZEST, size V stimulus
Ichhpujani et al., 2021	Visual Fields Easy (tablet based)	HFA, SITA Fast 24-2, size V stimulus
Johnson et al., 2017	Visual Fields Easy (tablet based)	HFA, SITA Standard 24-2, size V stimulus
Jones, 2020	Eye catcher (open-source eye-movement tracking perimeter)	HFA, SITA Standard 24-2, size III stimulus
Khizer et al., 2022	Specvic (computer-based)	HFA, SITA Standard 30-2, size III stimulus
Lam et al., 2017	Heidelberg Edge Perimeter	Octopus 900, G-TOP 30-2, size III stimulus

continued

TABLE 4-1 Continued

Citation	Index Test under Evaluation	Reference Standard
McLaughlin et al., 2023	Virtual Vision LCD VR visual field device	HFA, SITA analog, size III stimulus
Mees et al., 2020	C3 Fields Analyzer (head-mounted VR)	HFA, SITA Standard 24-2, 0.55 mm stimulus
Meyerov et al., 2023	Online Circular Contrast Perimetry (computer-based)	HFA, SITA analog, size III stimulus
Munshi et al., 2022	VR headset	HFA, SITA Standard 24-2, size III stimulus
Najdawi et al., 2023	Smart System VR Perimeter	HFA, SITA Standard 24-2, size III stimulus
Narang et al., 2021	Advanced Vision Analyzer VR perimeter	HFA, SITA Standard 24-2, size III stimulus
Olsen et al., 2017	Damato Multifixation Campimetry Online, an inexpensive online test	HFA, SITA Fast 30-2, stimulus size not reported
Pradhan et al., 2021	GearVision (smartphone-based, head-mounted Perimeter)	HFA, SITA Standard 24-2, size III stimulus
Schulz et al., 2018	Melbourne Rapid Fields (tablet based)	HFA, SITA Standard 24-2, size III stimulus
Susanna et al., 2024	VisuALL (VR head-mounted visual perimetry device)	HFA, SITA Fast 24-2, size III stimulus
Terracciano et al., 2023	Portable automatic kinetic perimeter based on a VR headset device	HFA, algorithm and stimulus size not reported
Tsapakis et al., 2018	Home (computer)-based visual field test for glaucoma screening	HFA, proprietary suprathreshold algorithm, size III stimulus
Tsiogka et al., 2024	TsiogkaSpaeth grid (portable test)	HFA, SITA Standard 24-2, size III stimulus
Vingrys et al., 2016	Melbourne Rapid Fields (tablet based)	HFA, SITA Standard 24-2, size V stimulus
Wijayagunaratne et al., 2023 (conference abstract)	Iowa Head Mounted Display perimeter	Octopus 900, standard algorithm, stimulus size not reported
Wroblewski et al., 2014	VirtualEye	HFA, SITA Standard or SITA Fast 24-2, size III stimulus

NOTES: The studies in the table were found in the committee's literature review of perimetry validation studies from 2002 to the present. Only studies with a reference standard were included in this table. Participants in the studies in the table were either glaucoma patients at various stages of the condition only, or glaucoma patients compared with controls. To identify perimetry validation studies, a search was conducted in Medline, Scopus, and Embase for ("visual field test*" OR perimetry) AND validat* in the title, abstract or keywords for articles published 2002 to the present. The search yielded 832 results after deduplicating, and 216 results after initial screening. These studies were then reviewed manually to identify those that aimed to validate a new perimeter and/or compare different perimeters, excluding those that focused on analysis of data from a single existing perimeter. HFA = Humphrey Field Analyzer; SITA = Swedish Interactive Thresholding Algorithm.

of participants is to be drawn. Another valid design for comparing two diagnostic tests is a randomized trial, where a group of eligible participants is assigned randomly to one of two diagnostic tests. The accuracy of the tests is then compared to evaluate their performance.

Diagnostic test accuracy studies sometimes include healthy controls or patients with a preexisting diagnosis without requiring all participants to undergo a reference test. These studies, known as "two-gate studies," use two or more sets of eligibility criteria, meaning both enrollment and later statistical comparison are based on disease status. This design was previously referred to as "diagnostic case-control" design.

The bias associated with the two-gate design primarily stems from the nonrandom selection of participants. Empirical evidence indicates that accuracy is overestimated in two-gate studies (Lijmer et al., 1999; Rutjes et al., 2006). This is so because as an alternative to enrolling a full spectrum of patients, use of the index test among the group with a preexisting diagnosis makes cases easier to detect, which leads to higher estimates of sensitivity. Likewise, the inclusion of healthy controls is likely to lower the occurrence of false-positive results, thereby increasing specificity. (Sensitivity and specificity are defined below.) In summary, when participant enrollment in a test accuracy study is conditional on disease status, the disease severity is likely to be at the extremes of the spectrum, raising similar concerns about spectrum bias.

To determine how much evidence or what type of evidence is sufficient to validate a new test, it is necessary to consider the quality of that evidence, often referred to as "risk of bias." QUADAS-2 is one widely accepted tool for assessing risk of bias in diagnostic test accuracy studies. Important contributors to the risk of bias include patient selection (see the above discussion of spectrum bias); potential differential verification if not all participants undergo both the index test and the reference test in the same way or at the time of the study; and whether the index test and reference test were conducted according to a predefined protocol, with results interpreted independently from each other (Whiting et al., 2011).

Finally, as noted earlier, it is important for diagnostic test accuracy studies to be conducted in a setting that accords with the intended setting of use. For example, if a test is assessed in a research setting with optimal test conditions and supervised by an expert technician, the results of the study may not apply to conduct of the test in the office of a primary care physician.

PERFORMANCE CONSIDERATIONS FOR EVALUATING NEW PERIMETRY TECHNIQUES

For a perimetry technique to assess disability effectively and accurately, its results must be valid, reliable, reproducible, and applicable for the specific task at hand. The critical question is whether the results are satisfactory according to four key considerations, based on the totality of evidence:

1. *Validity* refers to the ability of a perimetry technique to accurately identify whether an individual meets SSA's criteria for receiving disability benefits. Sensitivity and specificity are important metrics for assessing validity. Sensitivity measures the test's ability to correctly identify those with disability, while specificity measures its capacity to correctly identify those without it. Both sensitivity and specificity can be estimated only in a population that properly represents the target population (thus avoiding spectrum bias). Both sensitivity and specificity need to be measured with sufficient precision to permit confident evaluation against the SSA criteria, and this precision should be reported or at least be able to be calculated based on the reported information.
2. *Reliability indices*, as used in perimetry and in this report, are intended to indicate the confidence with which one can ascertain whether the results of a single test are credible or they require repetition or rejection. Perimetry reliability indices include the proportions of false-positive responses, false-negative responses, and fixation losses (defined later).
3. *Reproducibility* emphasizes the consistency of results across multiple tests, ensuring satisfactory test–retest consistency. Reproducibility is sometimes referred to as reliability in other diagnostic testing contexts, which can lead to confusion. In the context of this report, the committee distinguishes reproducibility as the degree to which results remain consistent (or less variable) over repeated measurements.
4. *Applicability* refers to the extent to which the results of a perimetry technique can be generalized to the target population and the setting for which the test is intended—in other words, whether the study's findings are relevant and applicable to the specific clinical context in which the test is meant to be used.

These four considerations can be addressed within a single study or across separate studies. Ideally for SSA's purposes, a perimetry technique would be evaluated in a way that aligns with its intended use and target population specifically in the context of determining whether an individual meets the criteria for visual field loss in connection with SSA disability evaluation (applicability). However, the committee's review of the literature revealed no studies that directly examined a perimetry technique for this specific purpose. In the absence of such studies, correlation with a reference standard perimeter in eyes with moderate and/or severe functional loss can be used as a proxy, as those types of studies *are* available in the literature (see Table 3-1).

Most studies in the literature focus explicitly on patients with glaucoma, as this is the most common population tested clinically using perimetry. Many of these studies examine the ability to classify eyes as healthy versus glaucomatous, which is of limited relevance to the ability to perform disability evaluation, especially given that reproducibility often declines as functional loss increases with advancing glaucoma (Artes et al., 2002).

Studies of perimetry for people with glaucoma may not fully reflect the pathology or visual experience of people with other ophthalmic disorders, such as those of the outer retina or cortex. The mean deviation or visual field may be similar in two individuals with each respective disease, but their eyesight as a whole may be very different. However, this report is primarily concerned with the evaluation of visual fields against the SSA criteria; other aspects of vision can be evaluated through other parts of the SSA disability determination process (see Chapter 1). In this context, the committee is comfortable extrapolating findings of visual field loss across diseases.

Validity

In general, validity refers to the ability of a test or protocol to actually capture what it intends to capture. As stated, the relevant definition of validity in this report is the ability of a perimetry technique to accurately identify whether an individual meets SSA's criteria for receiving disability benefits.

Sensitivity and specificity are important metrics for assessing validity. Since the key question examined in this report is how to feasibly determine whether an individual with visual field loss meets SSA's criteria for visual disability, permissible methods must necessarily have acceptable sensitivity and specificity. Simply assessing whether a test can classify eyes as "normal" or "abnormal" is inadequate. Instead, it is crucial to evaluate the test's ability to differentiate between "moderate" and "severe" visual field loss. While this distinction does not directly capture SSA's specific criteria for disability evaluation, eligibility depends on *how* severely a person's visual field is constricted (see Chapter 1). As a result, the most relevant studies will evaluate a perimetry test's ability to discern between *levels* of impairment. Additionally, considerations of validity encompass all domains related to risk of bias in diagnostic test accuracy studies, as outlined in the previous section and throughout this chapter.

Another relevant consideration is the measurement precision reported by the instrument, which affects the numerical range of outcomes that can possibly be reported. Typically, perimeters round visual field data to the nearest integer.

Reliability Indices

Test reliability in perimetry has traditionally been assessed using the three indices of false positives, false negatives, and fixation losses. While a new perimetry technique need not adhere strictly to this framework, not least because those indices are now not seen as particularly good measures of reliability, it is reasonable to consider whether equivalent information is available in a studied technique. Notably, poor reliability indices can hinder the detection and monitoring of small visual field defects; however, the committee felt that these indices may have less impact on mean deviation and assessment of current standards for visual disability. Mean deviation quantifies the degree to which a patient's visual sensitivity across the entire field differs from what is expected in a healthy individual of the same age.

False positives occur when an individual undergoing perimetry testing indicates they have seen a stimulus when none has been presented. This possibility can be assessed through catch trials, in which no stimulus is shown during an interval when one might be expected. If the examinee indicates seeing a stimulus during such an interval, this is considered a false-positive response. Additionally, false positives can be identified by recording responses that occur outside the physiologically plausible period of time after presentation of a stimulus. A high false-positive rate can be an indicator of "trigger-happy" behavior on the part of the patient, which may in turn lead to test results that do not accurately reflect the extent of visual field loss. Clinical guidelines often recommend that a test be considered unreliable if false-positive responses exceed 15 percent, though some test results with higher false-positive rates can still be useful (Heijl et al., 2021). This is because the impact of false positives on mean sensitivity is relatively minor; a 10-percentage-point increase in the false-positive rate has been estimated to raise mean deviation by 0.3–0.4 decibels (dB) in eyes with early-stage glaucoma, and by up to 1.4 dB in cases of severe glaucoma (Heijl et al., 2022).

False negatives occur when an individual being tested fails to respond to a stimulus that, based on the test as a whole, they should be able to see. In other words, a false negative is when an examinee fails to respond to a stimulus that is significantly higher in intensity than the patient's calculated threshold at that location. In damaged areas of the visual field, the frequency-of-seeing curve is very shallow (Gardiner et al., 2014). For example, a stimulus 6 dB more intense than the detection threshold[2] may still go unnoticed, even by a perfectly reliable observer (Gardiner et al., 2014). As a result, the frequency of false-negative responses tends to reflect the status of the disease more than the reliability of the test itself (Bengtsson and Heijl, 2000).

---

[2] As discussed in Chapter 3, the standard unit for measuring the visual field is differential light sensitivity, which defines the threshold for detecting a test object relative to its background.

While the committee felt that the false-negative index remains useful in certain circumstances, a high false-negative rate does not necessarily mean that a test should be discounted entirely. For example, a visual field with greater than 33 percent false negatives may be acceptable if other clinical information supports the presence of severe loss of vision.

Fixation refers to the process of maintaining the gaze on a specific point or target in the visual field. In the context of visual field testing, it usually involves keeping the eyes steady on a designated fixation point while stimuli are presented in the surrounding areas. Traditionally, fixation losses have been evaluated using catch trials. At the beginning of the test, the perimeter maps the position of the blind spot. Stimuli are then presented in that region; if the examinee responds, it is recorded as a fixation loss. A test is typically considered unreliable if an individual responds to more than 20 percent of these catch trials (Heijl et al., 2012). However, this assessment can be inaccurate if the blind spot is incorrectly mapped at the outset. Assessment also becomes challenging during binocular visual field testing with both eyes open unless the stimulus can be directed to just one eye—possible with a virtual reality headset but not with tablets or personal computer screens. Moreover, tests in which the fixation target is not central can lead to greater loss of fixation, reducing the reliability of the test results. For example, when the fixation target is presented in the corner of the screen during perimetry testing using a tablet to increase the testable area, the location where the stimulus will appear relative to the target point is within a much narrower range of the visual field than when the testing uses a bowl perimeter device. Thus, the individual being tested may tend to move their gaze in the direction in which the stimulus is expected to appear.

An approach newer than catch trials involves using a built-in camera for fixation monitoring, which may offer equivalent or improved accuracy. A trace of fixation (a visual depiction of where an individual's gaze was focused during the test) can be a useful tool for educating the patient, as well as a useful indicator of poor test reliability. However, the fixation trace must be quantified before an appropriate threshold can be established. Gaze-tracking measurements do not always correlate well with the probability of fixation losses (Camp et al., 2022), and it remains unclear which method is superior for assessing test reliability. (See Figure 3-6 [j] in Chapter 3 for an example of how variability in gaze during a perimetry test is reported.) Furthermore, head position tracking does not provide equivalent information, as it may not detect fixation movements.

Poor fixation can result in missed localized defects, as well as inaccuracies in measuring their spatial extent or depth. However, the committee notes that the impact on global averages, such as mean deviation, is smaller; excessive fixation losses have been shown to have only a minor effect on mean deviation (Yohannan et al., 2017). Poor fixation could cause the patient to observe and respond to stimuli that they would not otherwise have seen, reducing the apparent severity of the defect; this is a critical problem when, for example, assessing the ability to drive. However, the committee agreed that it would be very unlikely to cause an overestimate of defect severity to a degree that would impede accurate disability assessment.

Given these caveats regarding reliability indices, it is not always appropriate to treat them as fixed binary cutoffs. Instead, it is best to examine a test result that appears to have poor reliability to determine why poor reliability indices were measured. For example, a high false-negative rate might be caused by low visual sensitivity. Given such an explanation, the test result may still provide sufficient information for the assessment of disability. At the same time, the committee was unable to find literature supporting specific alternatives that could be used as guidelines or cutoffs instead of reliability indices. As a result, the committee instead notes that the results of a perimetry test need to be analyzed holistically. In other words, evaluating a new perimetry technique requires more than simply assessing the result of its validation studies. It is also important to examine the metrics those validation studies use to judge a technique reliable or unreliable.

It is therefore advisable to collect and report reliability indices, as these are an essential piece of information to be included in that assessment.

Reproducibility

Interpretation of test reproducibility is best carried out in the context of the severity of visual field loss. The most commonly used static automated threshold perimetry test in the United States employs a 24-2 testing pattern using the SITA Standard testing algorithm, modulating stimulus contrast with a Goldmann size III stimulus, on a Humphrey Field Analyzer perimeter. When a location appears healthy (sensitivity 30–35 dB), the measured sensitivity upon retesting that same location typically varies with a standard deviation of ±1 dB (Artes et al., 2002). Test–retest variability increases with greater visual field loss. For locations with sensitivity of 10–15 dB (around the mean deviation cutoff of 22 dB or greater for visual disability by current SSA standards), the standard deviation for test–retest variability rises to ±6 dB (Artes et al., 2002). For intensities brighter than 15–20 dB, the probability of responding to the stimulus plateaus, meaning further increases in brightness have minimal impact on detectability, which hinders accurate measurement of severe visual field loss (Gardiner et al., 2014).

Variability in results may also arise from different levels of contrast. Research has shown that testing with contrasts greater than 15–20 dB on a

Humphrey Field Analyzer does not enhance the ability to detect progression and can be excluded without loss of information (Gardiner et al., 2016; Wall et al., 2018). Although SSA's current standards for visual disability indicate the ability to detect a stimulus corresponding to 10-dB contrast on a Humphrey Field Analyzer, it is likely that equivalent results can be achieved using a stimulus corresponding to a 15-dB contrast.

Alternative perimetry techniques can yield varying metrics that influence reproducibility. For example, using a larger stimulus size generally increases mean sensitivities and reduces variability. Additionally, different types of stimuli may exhibit distinct variability profiles. Testing algorithms may adjust stimulus size or other characteristics in addition to, or instead of, modifying intensity, and results may be expressed in units other than dB.

A benchmark for reproducibility is whether test results from the perimetry technique being evaluated are as reproducible as those from the current clinical standard. In this context, the relevant metric is the probability that a patient would continue to meet SSA's criteria for visual disability if they met those criteria the previous day, regardless of whether the same or a different test was used, and whether this probability is similar to that of the current benchmark. If necessary, disability criteria or guides to their interpretations could be modified to reflect the equivalent criteria from current clinical standard testing. When assessing a new perimetry technique, a primary consideration is comparing the intertechnique variability (i.e., between two tests conducted with different perimeters) against the intratechnique variability (i.e., between two tests conducted with the current clinical standard perimeter), with a sufficiently short time between same- or different-technique tests that there will have been no significant change in the patient's true level of visual function.

Applicability

Applicability considerations include such factors as the age, linguistic ability, and socioeconomic status of the study population, ensuring that they reflect those of the target population (see the earlier discussion of spectrum bias). For example, in the context of using perimetry to assess visual field defects for disability evaluation, the study population should represent the demographic characteristics of individuals who are undergoing SSA disability assessments. Based on this, all studies in Table 4-1 would be rated as having low applicability to SSA disability assessments. Additionally, it is important that the perimetry test used in the study closely mirrors the one that would be employed in real-world clinical settings. Differences in the test's procedure, technology, or interpretation—such as variations in testing protocols or the equipment used—could influence the generalizability of the study's findings to the target population.

QUANTITY AND CHARACTERISTICS OF VALIDATION STUDIES NEEDED TO FIND A PERIMETER ACCEPTABLE

The committee's statement of task asks whether three published clinical validation studies are needed to find a perimeter acceptable, and if fewer studies are acceptable, what the requirements of the study design would be.

If the instrument or software is expected to be used in diverse populations or clinical settings, having more studies can help demonstrate its validity, reliability, and applicability across different conditions. More studies can provide a larger sample size, which may improve the statistical power and robustness of the findings. However, the committee's judgment is that the quality, relevance, and totality of the evidence are more important than the number of studies available. Therefore, the committee concluded that it is not possible to quantify the number of studies required to find a perimetry technique acceptable, and accordingly, this chapter does not stipulate a required number of published studies. Instead, it highlights essential factors to be considered when considering whether a study evaluating a new perimetry technique is well designed.[3] Such studies need to address clinically relevant endpoints and demonstrate how the new technique compares with existing standards. In the case of vision-related disability, it will be important to ensure that the combination of the hardware and software measures the boundaries of the visual field requirements outlined by SSA.

SUMMARY AND CONCLUSIONS

Validating a new perimetry technique requires a thorough assessment of its validity, reliability indices, reproducibility, and applicability, all aligned with its intended use in SSA disability evaluation. The ideal study assessing a new perimetry technique is designed in a way that directly evaluates its intended use and target population—for this report, specifically to determine whether an individual meets the criteria for visual field loss in connection with SSA disability evaluation. Given that the committee's review of the literature revealed no studies that directly examined a perimetry technique for this specific purpose, one could use correlation with a reference standard perimeter in eyes with moderate and/or severe functional loss as a proxy. As reference standards are typically the current "gold standard," comparing new perimeters with the Humphrey Field Analyzer using a size III stimulus may generate useful evidence.

---

[3] Regulatory bodies such as the Food and Drug Administration (FDA) in the United States may have specific guidelines regarding the number and type of studies required for validation. In addition, FDA and other federal agencies have encouraged a patient-centered outcomes approach for assessing the functionality and effectiveness of devices.

Determination of the acceptability of a new perimetry technique needs to focus on the specific combination of hardware, stimuli, testing patterns, and algorithms, not solely on the device itself. Also essential is to take the scope of evidence into account, including data from diverse populations and real-world settings, to ensure that the technique performs effectively across patients with various underlying clinical conditions. Two well-designed, adequately powered studies may provide more reliable evidence than three poorly designed ones.

To determine how much or what type of evidence is sufficient, one must also consider the quality of the information, often referred to as risk of bias. QUADAS-2 is one widely accepted tool for assessing risk of bias in diagnostic test accuracy studies. Important contributors to risk of bias include potential differential verification; patient selection; and whether the index test and reference test were conducted according to a predefined protocol, with results interpreted independently.

Based on its review of the literature and the committee's expert assessment, the committee reached the following conclusions:

Conclusion 4.1: When assessing the acceptability of a technique for visual field assessment, the quality, relevance, and totality of the evidence are more important than the number of published studies available.

Conclusion 4.2: Sensitivity (in the sense of a test's ability to identify correctly those with a qualifying disability) and specificity (a test's capacity to identify correctly those without a qualifying disability) are important metrics for assessing a test's internal validity. Both specificity and sensitivity need to be measured with sufficient precision to permit confident evaluation against the SSA criteria.

Based on its review of the literature, the committee reached the following conclusion:

Conclusion 4.3: Test results that appear to have poor reliability indices need to be examined to determine whether the results may still be useful for identifying deficits that qualify for disability benefits by providing sufficient information for the determination of disability.

With intensities above 15–20 dB on a Humphrey Field Analyzer, or the equivalent on other instruments, the probability that an examinee will respond to the stimulus plateaus. Therefore, further increases in brightness have minimal impact on detectability, which hinders accurate measurement of severe field loss. Variability in results may also arise from different levels of contrast. Research has shown that testing with contrasts greater than 15–20 dB does not enhance the ability to detect progression of visual field impairment and can be excluded without loss of information.

Based on its review of the literature and the committee's expert assessment, the committee reached the following conclusion:

Conclusion 4.4: Although SSA's current criteria for visual disability require the ability to detect a stimulus corresponding to 10-dB contrast on a Humphrey Field Analyzer perimeter, it is likely that equivalent results can be achieved using a stimulus corresponding to a 15-dB contrast.

REFERENCES

Ahmed, Y., A. Pereira, S. Bowden, R. B. Shi, Y. Li, I. I. K. Ahmed, and S. A. Arshinoff. 2022. Multicenter comparison of the Toronto portable perimeter with the Humphrey Field Analyzer: A pilot study. *Ophthalmology Glaucoma* 5(2):146–159.

Artes, P. H., A. Iwase, Y. Ohno, Y. Kitazawa, and B. C. Chauhan. 2002. Properties of perimetric threshold estimates from full threshold, SITA standard, and SITA fast strategies. *Investigative Ophthalmology & Visual Science* 43(8):2654–2659.

Balasubramanian, G., J. C. Park, R. A. Hyde, and J. J. McAnany. 2023. Validation of a novel LED-based chromatic visual field perimeter. *Investigative Ophthalmology & Visual Science* 64(8):5344.

Bengtsson, B., and A. Heijl. 2000. False-negative responses in glaucoma perimetry: Indicators of patient performance or test reliability? *Investigative Ophthalmology & Visual Science* 41(8):2201–2204.

Bentley, S. A., R. P. LeBlanc, M. T. Nicolela, and B. C. Chauhan. 2012. Validity, reliability, and repeatability of the useful field of view test in persons with normal vision and patients with glaucoma. *Investigative Ophthalmology & Visual Science* 53(11):6763–6769.

Bradley, C., I. I. K. Ahmed, T. W. Samuelson, M. Chaglasian, H. Barnebey, N. Radcliffe, and J. Bacharach. 2024. Validation of a wearable virtual reality perimeter for glaucoma staging, the NOVA trial: Novel virtual reality field assessment. *Translational Vision & Science Technology* 13(3):10.

Camp, A. S., C. P. Long, V. M. Patella, J. A. Proudfoot, and R. N. Weinreb. 2022. Standard reliability and gaze tracking metrics in glaucoma and glaucoma suspects. *American Journal of Ophthalmology* 234:91–98.

Chen, Y. T., P. H. Yeh, Y. C. Cheng, W. W. Su, Y. S. Hwang, H. S. L. Chen, Y. S. Lee, and S. C. Shen. 2022. Application and validation of LUXIE: A newly developed virtual reality perimetry software. *Journal of Personalized Medicine* 12(10).

Chen, Z., X. Shen, Y. Zhang, W. Yang, J. Ye, Z. Ouyang, G. Zheng, Y. Yang, and M. Yu. 2024. Development and validation of an internet-based remote perimeter (Perimouse). *Translational Vision Science & Technology* 13(3):16.

Chia, M., A. Turner, G. Kong, A. Agar, and E. Trang. 2019. Validation of an iPad visual field test to screen for glaucoma in rural and remote settings. *Clinical and Experimental Ophthalmology* 47(Supplement 1):121.

Chia, M. A., E. Trang, A. Agar, A. J. Vingrys, J. Hepschke, G. Y. X. Kong, and A. W. Turner. 2021. Screening for glaucomatous visual field defects in rural Australia with an iPad. *Journal of Current Glaucoma Practice* 15(3):125–131.

Crossland, M. D., V. A. Luong, G. S. Rubin, and F. W. Fitzke. 2011. Retinal specific measurement of dark-adapted visual function: Validation of a modified microperimeter. *BMC Ophthalmology* 11:5.

Cui, Q. N., P. Gogt, J. M. Lam, S. Siraj, L. A. Hark, J. S. Myers, L. J. Katz, and M. Waisbourd. 2019. Validation and reproducibility of the Heidelberg edge perimeter in the detection of glaucomatous visual field defects. *International Journal of Ophthalmology* 12(4):577–581.

Deeks, J. J., P. M. Bossuyt, M. M. Leeflang, and Y. Takwoingi (Eds). 2023. *Cochrane handbook for systematic reviews of diagnostic test accuracy*, 1st ed. Chichester (UK): Wiley.

Gardiner, S. K., W. H. Swanson, and S. Demirel. 2016. The effect of limiting the range of perimetric sensitivities on pointwise assessment of visual field progression in glaucoma. *Investigative Ophthalmology & Visual Science* 57(1):288–294.

Gardiner, S. K., W. H. Swanson, D. Goren, S. L. Mansberger, and S. Demirel. 2014. Assessment of the reliability of standard automated perimetry in regions of glaucomatous damage. *Ophthalmology* 121(7):1359–1369.

Heijl, A., V. M. Patella, and B. Bengtsson. 2012. *The field analyzer primer: Effective perimetry*. Dublin, CA: Carl Zeiss Meditec, Inc.

Heijl, A., V. M. Patella, and B. Bengtsson. 2021. *The field analyzer primer: Excellent perimetry*, 5th edition. Carl Zeiss Meditec, Inc.

Heijl, A., V. M. Patella, J. G. Flanagan, A. Iwase, C. K. Leung, A. Tuulonen, G. C. Lee, T. Callan, and B. Bengtsson. 2022. False positive responses in standard automated perimetry. *American Journal of Ophthalmology* 233:180–188.

Heinzman, Z., K. Alawa, I. Marin-Franch, A. Turpin, and M. Wall. 2022. Validation of visual field results of a new open-source virtual reality headset. *Investigative Ophthalmology & Visual Science* 63(7):1259–A0399.

Heinzman, Z., E. Linton, I. Marín-Franch, A. Turpin, K. Alawa, A. Wijayagunaratne, and M. Wall. 2023. Validation of the Iowa head-mounted open-source perimeter. *Translational Vision Science & Technology* 12(9):19.

Ichhpujani, P., S. Thakur, R. K. Sahi, and S. Kumar. 2021. Validating tablet perimetry against standard Humphrey visual field analyzer for glaucoma screening in Indian population. *Indian Journal of Ophthalmology* 69(1):87–91.

Johnson, C. A., S. Thapa, Y. X. George Kong, and A. L. Robin. 2017. Performance of an iPad application to detect moderate and advanced visual field loss in Nepal. *American Journal of Ophthalmology* 182:147–154.

Jones, P. R. 2020. An open-source static threshold perimetry test using remote eye-tracking (eyecatcher): Description, validation, and preliminary normative data. *Translational Vision Science & Technology* 9(8):18.

Khizer, M. A., T. A. Khan, U. Ijaz, S. Khan, A. K. Rehmatullah, I. Zahid, H. G. Shah, M. A. Zahid, H. Sarfaraz, and N. Khurshid. 2022. Personal computer-based visual field testing as an alternative to standard automated perimetry. *Cureus* 14(12):e32094.

Lam, J. M., L. A. Hark, J. S. Myers, L. J. Katz, S. Siraj, M. Waisbourd, P. Gogte, and Q. J. Cui. 2017. Validation and reproducibility of the Heidelberg edge perimeter in the detection of visual field defects in glaucoma participants. *Investigative Ophthalmology & Visual Science* 58(8).

Lijmer, J. G., B. W. Mol, S. Heisterkamp, G. J. Bonsel, M. H. Prins, J. H. van der Meulen, and P. M. Bossuyt. 1999. Empirical evidence of design-related bias in studies of diagnostic tests. *JAMA* 282(11):1061–1066. https://doi.org/10.1001/jama.282.11.1061

McLaughlin, M., N. E. M. Sanal-Hayes, L. D. Hayes, E. C. Berry, and N. F. Sculthorpe. 2023. People with long COVID and myalgic encephalomyelitis/chronic fatigue syndrome exhibit similarly impaired vascular function. *American Journal of Medicine* 138(3):560–566.

Mees, L., S. Upadhyaya, P. Kumar, S. Kotawala, S. Haran, S. Rajasekar, D. S. Friedman, and R. Venkatesh. 2020. Validation of a head-mounted virtual reality visual field screening device. *Journal of Glaucoma* 29(2):86–91.

Meyerov, J., Y. Deng, L. Busija, D. Bigirimana, and S. E. Skalicky. 2023. Online circular contrast perimetry: A comparison to standard automated perimetry. *Asia-Pacific Journal of Ophthalmology* 12(1):4–15.

Munshi, H., K. Da Silva, E. Savatovsky, E. Bitrian, A. L. Grajewski, and T. C. Chang. 2022. Preliminary retrospective validation of a novel virtual reality visual field standard testing algorithm, as compared to standard automated perimetry. *Investigative Ophthalmology & Visual Science* 63(7):1275–A0415.

Najdawi, W., C. A. Johnson, and A. Pouw. 2023. Validation of a novel head-mounted perimeter versus the Humphrey Field Analyzer. *Investigative Ophthalmology & Visual Science* 64(8):5496.

Narang, P., A. Agarwal, M. Srinivasan, and A. Agarwal. 2021. Advanced vision analyzer-virtual reality perimeter: Device validation, functional correlation and comparison with Humphrey Field Analyzer. *Ophthalmology Science* 1(2):100035.

Olsen, A. S., A. T. Steensberg, M. la Cour, T. W. Kjaer, B. Damato, L. H. Pinborg, and M. Kolko. 2017. Can DMCO detect visual field loss in neurological patients? A secondary validation study. *Ophthalmic Research* 58(2):85–93.

Pradhan, Z. S., T. Sircar, H. Agrawal, H. L. Rao, A. Bopardikar, S. Devi, and V. N. Tiwari. 2021. Comparison of the performance of a novel, smartphone-based, head-mounted perimeter (Gearvision) with the Humphrey Field Analyzer. *Journal of Glaucoma* 30(4):E146–E152.

Rutjes, A. W., J. B. Reitsma, M. Di Nisio, N. Smidt, J. C. van Rijn, and P. M. Bossuyt. 2006. Evidence of bias and variation in diagnostic accuracy studies. *Canadian Medical Association* 174(4):469–476.

Schulz, A. M., E. C. Graham, Y. You, A. Klistorner, and S. L. Graham. 2018. Performance of iPad-based threshold perimetry in glaucoma and controls. *Clinical & Experimental Ophthalmology* 46(4):346–355.

Susanna, F. N., C. N. Susanna, P. G. Salomão Libânio, F. T. Nishikawa, R. A. Schiave Germano, and R. S. Junior. 2024. Comparison between the fast strategies of a virtual reality perimetry and the Humphrey Field Analyzer in patients with glaucoma. *Ophthalmology Glaucoma*, S2589–4196(24):00219-9.

Terracciano, R., A. Mascolo, L. Venturo, F. Guidi, M. Vaira, C. M. Eandi, and D. Demarchi. 2023. Kinetic perimetry on virtual reality headset. *IEEE Transactions on Biomedical Circuits and Systems* 17(3):413–419.

Tsapakis, S., D. Papaconstantinou, A. Diagourtas, S. Kandarakis, K. Droutsas, K. Andreanos, and D. Brouzas. 2018. Home-based visual field test for glaucoma screening comparison with Humphrey perimeter. *Clinical Ophthalmology* 12:2597–2606.

Tsiogka, A., M. L. Moster, K. I. Chatzistefanou, E. Karmiris, E. Samoli, I. Giachos, K. Droutsas, D. Papaconstantinou, and G. L. Spaeth. 2024. The TsiogkaSpaeth grid for detection of neurological visual field defects: a validation study. *Neurological Sciences* 45(6):2869–2875.

Vingrys, A. J., J. K. Healey, S. Liew, V. Saharinen, M. Tran, W. Wu, and G. Y. Kong. 2016. Validation of a tablet as a tangent perimeter. *Translational Vision Science & Technology* 5(4):3.

Wall, M., G. K. D. Zamba, and P. H. Artes. 2018. The effective dynamic ranges for glaucomatous visual field progression with standard automated perimetry and stimulus sizes III and V. *Investigative Ophthalmology & Visual Science* 59(1):439–445.

Whiting, P. F., A. W. Rutjes, M. E. Westwood, S. Mallett, J. J. Deeks, J. B. Reitsma, M. M. Leeflang, J. A. Sterne, and P. M. Bossuyt. 2011. QUADAS-2: A revised tool for the quality assessment of diagnostic accuracy studies. *Annals of Internal Medicine* 155(8):529–536.

Wijayagunaratne, A., E. Linton, I. M. Franch, K. Alawa, and M. Wall. 2023. Smartphone perimetry: Comparison to standard automated perimetry and assessment of size-modulation strategy with frequency-of-seeing curves in healthy subjects. *Investigative Ophthalmology & Visual Science* 64(8):1502.

Wroblewski, D., B. A. Francis, A. Sadun, G. Vakili, and V. Chopra. 2014. Testing of visual field with virtual reality goggles in manual and visual grasp modes. *BioMed Research International* 2014:206082.

Yohannan, J., J. Wang, J. Brown, B. C. Chauhan, M. V. Boland, D. S. Friedman, and P. Y. Ramulu. 2017. Evidence-based criteria for assessment of visual field reliability. *Ophthalmology* 124(11):1612–1620.

5

Special Topics

The Social Security Administration (SSA) asked the committee to address several special topics in perimetry that pertain primarily to the acceptability of various technologies and techniques for assessing visual field loss for disability determination:

- Is optical projection of the testing stimuli still necessary to achieve valid and reliable results from a perimeter?
- How does the eye respond differently to projected versus other types of stimuli (e.g., liquid-crystal display [LCD] screens)?
- Do perimeters using frequency doubling technology produce results substantially similar to those obtained with traditional perimeters, and what differences are there?
- Is semiautomated kinetic perimetry a valid and reliable method of measuring visual field loss? What are the necessary device specifications and testing circumstances for semiautomated kinetic perimetry to produce valid and reliable visual field testing?
- What are the most widely acceptable and commonly used alternatives to kinetic perimetry, both manual and automated, for the measurement of visual field efficiency?
- What impacts do such alternative methods have on the validity and reliability of testing results?

This chapter also contains a section highlighting special considerations for evaluating perimetry in children. When developing perimetry guidelines, understanding differences related to pediatric versus adult populations is crucial because visual field testing in children presents unique challenges and requires age-appropriate strategies. Additionally, tailoring perimetric approaches to a child's specific developmental stage and cognitive ability ensures more reliable and informative results. This context is essential for accurately determining the role and interpretation of perimetry in children.

OPTICAL PROJECTION VERSUS SCREEN-BASED STIMULI

Across the Special Senses and Speech listings (SSA, n.d.), current SSA perimetric requirements specify the use of a white size III Goldmann stimulus against a 31.5-apostilb or 10-candela-per-square-meter (cd/m^2) white background. Recent developments in perimetry, however, have included new ways to present stimuli. These include desk-based instruments that utilize screen-based stimuli (e.g., Tempo), smartphones, tablets, and virtual reality (VR) headsets. Screens on these devices use either LCDs or organic light-emitting diode (OLED) microdisplays. LCDs use passive backlit illumination, while OLED displays use active illumination.

Screen-based perimeters are typically smaller than traditional perimeters and are based on technology available to consumers at lower prices. They may therefore be cheaper, although screen-based perimeters are a relatively new technology and so at present may still be expensive. Since these perimeters are similar to consumer technology, examinees may find them easier to use than traditional perimeters. Some studies have found that acceptability for VR-based perimeters is similar to or better than that for traditional perimeters (Ahmed et al., 2022; Wroblewski et al., 2014). While some individuals may not be familiar with them, evidence also suggests that people can feasibly be trained to complete perimetry examinations successfully with VR headsets (Chia et al., 2024).

One potential downside of screen-based perimeters is that screens rely on pixelation, or the creation of images from an aggregate of individual, small points of light. This may introduce technical limitations for the presentation of perimetric stimuli. For example, a screen cannot illuminate an image smaller than the size of the pixels supported by that screen (typically, the size of an individual diode or LCD crystal). Similarly, a screen may not be able to display a perfectly circular stimulus, depending on the pixel size. However, if demonstrated to be valid and reliable with respect to disability classification tasks, these stimuli could be used in place of optical projection for visual field testing.

Effect of Stimulus Luminance on Vision

To increase the possible contrast between background and stimulus, background luminance has been lowered for some screen-based devices.

SPECIAL TOPICS

Table 5-1 summarizes the luminance of the backgrounds and stimuli used in both standard and a selection of novel perimeters.

Table 5-1 is not intended to be a complete list of the screen-based perimeters currently being developed or used; rather, it is meant to illustrate the considerable variance in parameters across such devices. Some perimeters also have unique design features. For example, Vivid Vision and C3 perform suprathreshold tests, which present stimuli significantly brighter than the expected threshold of visual detection. In other words, these stimuli can be expected to always be seen by a person of the patient's age.

TABLE 5-1 Summary of Stimuli in Standard and Selected Novel Perimeters

Device Name	Type	Background Luminance	Maximum Luminance	Stimulus Used
Humphrey Field Analyzer 3	Standard	10 cd/m^2	3,183 cd/m^2	Variable
Octopus 900	Standard	1.27–10.00 cd/m^2	1,260 cd/m^2	Variable
Oculus	VR	10 cd/m^2	88 cd/m^2	Goldmann size III
SmartCampiTracker	Smartphone	0.05 cd/m^2	500 cd/m^2	Goldmann size III
Toronto Portable Perimeter	VR	10 cd/m^2	NR	Goldmann size III, IV, or V
Virtual Eye	OLED VR	NR	NR	Goldmann size III
Advanced Vision Analyzer	VR	9.6 cd/m^2	NR	Goldmann size III
Olleyes VisuALL	VR	1–3 cd/m^2	120 cd/m^2	Goldmann size III
Vivid Vision	VR	25 cd/m^2	NR[a]	Goldmann size III (black)
C3 Field Analyzer	VR	4 cd/m^2	NR[b]	Goldmann size III
Virtual Field	VR	0.218 cd/m^2	87 cd/m^2	0.55-mm circular stimuli
Radius	VR	10 cd/m^2	85 cd/m^2	Goldmann size II and III
TEMPO	Tabletop binocular	10 cd/m^2	3,183 cd/m^2	Variable (Goldmann size I through >V)

[a] In contrast to most screen-based perimeters, the Vivid Vision perimeter presents small black spots of luminance 0.2 cd/m^2 against a white background, rather than brighter white spots against a white background.
[b] Stimuli brightness was set at 60 cd/m^2.
NOTES: Some articles reported using a stimulus size of 0.43°, which is equivalent to Goldmann size III. NR = not reported; OLED = organic LED; VR = virtual reality.
SOURCES: Ahmed et al. (2022); Berneshawi et al. (2024); Bradley et al. (2024); Chia et al. (2024); Grau et al. (2023); Greenfield et al. (2022); Grobbel et al. (2016); Mees et al. (2020); Narang et al. (2021); Phu et al. (2025); Razeghinejad et al. (2021); Stapelfeldt et al. (2021); Topcon Healthcare (2025); Wroblewski et al. (2014).

Suprathreshold tests are generally used as screening tests or in settings where a complete field cut (an area of blindness) is expected. Vivid Vision also employs a black stimulus on a white background. The Advanced Vision Analyzer and Virtual Field devices include built-in hardware to allow for the use of trial lenses, while the Olleyes VisuALL allows examinees to wear their own glasses, though bifocals and trifocals are not recommended for use alongside this perimeter due to possible effects on retinal sensitivity. Finally, many of these devices, especially the VR-based platforms, include fixation tracking.

Note that many novel screen-based perimeters are unable to achieve the same range of luminance as traditional perimeters. However, in theory, similar relative brightnesses can still be achieved between the background and stimulus luminance, allowing for measurement against the SSA criteria. To be able to do so, the perimeter must be able to present a contrast equivalent to 10 decibels (dB) (in turn corresponding to approximately 22 dB of sensitivity loss if the respondent cannot see it) on the Humphrey Field Analyzer. In other words, it must be equivalent to a stimulus luminance of 318 cd/m^2 against a 10 cd/m^2 background on the Humphrey Field Analyzer. A lower maximum stimulus intensity may be adequate if the background luminance is reduced; however, the background must still be of sufficient luminance to remain within the photopic range of sight.[1] Not all of the perimeters in Table 5-1 meet both these requirements, but more may be developed in the future.

Changes in stimulus size can also be made equivalent to changes in stimulus intensity. Whether a stimulus is perceived or not depends on the number of photons stimulating the retina and the area of the retina being stimulated. The likelihood of perception can be increased by increasing either stimulus intensity or stimulus size. Some testing protocols, such as the protocol used by the Toronto Portable Perimeter, involve using a larger stimulus size to test lower-threshold sensitivity (Ahmed et al., 2022), although the data on this change in stimulus size are still emerging. A more detailed discussion of the effect of stimulus size can be found later in this chapter.

It is also necessary to consider that perimetric data are conventionally reported in decibels, which is a measure of stimulus luminance relative to the maximum that can be produced in a specific device. A higher decibel value reflects greater attenuation, or dimming, of the eye's ability to perceive stimuli. If two devices use different background luminances, use of the same stimulus luminance on these different devices will result in a different contrast. Thus, decibel measurements produced by devices with different luminances may not be directly comparable (Phu et al., 2025). However, if the luminosity, background, perceived color, and size of a stimulus are all

---

[1] This sentence was changed after release of the report to correct the description of the range of sight.

held equal, that stimulus should be seen similarly by the eye regardless of whether the stimulus is projected or displayed on a screen, as long as the background luminance is within the limits of Weber's law. In other words, in photopic light conditions, the smallest noticeable difference between two stimuli will be proportional to the original stimulus's intensity, not a constant absolute difference. Under less luminant mesopic conditions, Weber's law does not hold, but because standard methods of perimetry are performed under photopic conditions, this concern should not affect disability determination. Screen-based perimeters can strengthen this consistency by accurately measuring and reporting these metrics.

Luminance changes can cause people to use the mesopic range of vision (0.01–3.00 cd/m^2) rather than the photopic range (>3.00 cd/m^2). Both rods and cones are active in the mesopic range, while only cones are active in the photopic range (Bradley et al., 2024).[2] The direct clinical significance of this nuance in evaluating visual field loss is currently unclear for people with glaucoma, but this can have marked effects in patients lacking rod function, as these patients may use cones only at conditions that would otherwise be in the mesopic or high scotopic range. Similarly, people who are color-blind or otherwise lacking cone function may also be affected differentially by changes in luminance. When performing perimetry tests in both of these populations, examiners need to be aware of how different light levels may affect their results.

For the purposes of identifying visual field loss as part of disability determination, clinical validation data for newer testing platforms relevant to SSA criteria for visual disability are more important than strict requirements based on stimulus type (i.e., projected versus nonprojected). Other differences in devices (e.g., background luminance, black versus white stimulus, colored stimuli) are of little importance if the validity and reproducibility of the clinical test results are demonstrated.

Conclusions

A strong and growing body of literature supports the acceptable clinical performance of perimeters that do not use optical stimulus projection. While theoretically the perception of projected and nonprojected stimuli that are otherwise similar should be the same, scientific evidence specifically evaluating the consistency of testing results using different types of stimuli is limited. Future clinical studies may fill this gap in the literature.

Screen-based perimeters may become more acceptable and reliable for the average patient, as they are both cheaper than traditional perimeters

---

[2] Rods are the cells in the retina that are sensitive to low-light conditions and are responsible for night vision. Cones are the cells that are sensitive to bright light and are responsible for color vision and seeing fine detail.

and based on common consumer electronics. VR perimeters, in particular, may be able to include eye tracking and ensure fixation, which would increase their reliability. As these technologies develop, allowing their use for SSA disability determination would make perimetry easier, more available, and less costly for more people.

At the same time, however, these new technologies come with substantial uncertainties in performance. Luminance varies significantly between different screen-based perimeters, and stimuli may not be exactly the same as in traditional perimeters because of limitations in modern screen-based technology. Many screen-based perimeters are also not able to achieve the range of luminance (especially at the dim end) that is achieved in table-top perimeters.

Device manufacturers can mitigate these challenges in a variety of ways, such as by modifying the stimulus intensity, size, and duration. Different test patterns may also be feasible in the future. In theory, variations in these design factors could result in stimuli that are functionally equivalent to those presented by traditional perimeters. As discussed in Chapter 4, effective validation of these novel technologies for use in SSA disability determination would likely involve comparing their performance on classification tasks directly to that of currently accepted projection-based methods.

Based on its review of the evidence and the committee's expert assessment, the committee reached the following conclusions:

Conclusion 5.1: The technology used to present stimuli and backgrounds during perimetry, such as optical projection or video screens, is unlikely to have a substantial effect on visual perception or test results. However, because perimeters using nonprojected visuals have been developed only relatively recently, evaluation studies of such perimeters will be most useful if they robustly report specific testing parameters and the technical details of the device.

Conclusion 5.2: The suitability of novel perimeters for SSA's use in disability determination is affected by their performance relative to that of current methods; comparative validation studies, ideally using SSA-relevant classification tasks, will therefore be the best way to assess suitability.

FREQUENCY DOUBLING TECHNOLOGY

Frequency doubling technology (FDT), or frequency doubling perimetry, has been used for decades, primarily as a screening device for visual impairment in the community. As in static automated threshold perimetry (SAP) protocols, FDT entails asking examinees to fixate on a central point and indicate when they see a stimulus beyond that point. The patient indicates when they perceive the flickering stimulus, and the system records these responses. Areas where the patient fails to detect the stimulus indicate potential visual field loss.

Unlike SAP, FDT presents a pattern of alternating light and dark bars called a "sinusoidal grating." This grating is typically set at a specific spatial frequency (e.g., 0.25 cycles per degree). The key feature of the stimulus is that it is flickered at a high temporal frequency (usually around 25 hertz [Hz]; see Figure 5-1). The visual system perceives this as a single pulse of light flickering at twice the true spatial frequency, an effect known as frequency doubling. Differences in examinees' sensitivity to these stimuli are therefore related to the frequency of this flickering, not the luminance of the stimulus.

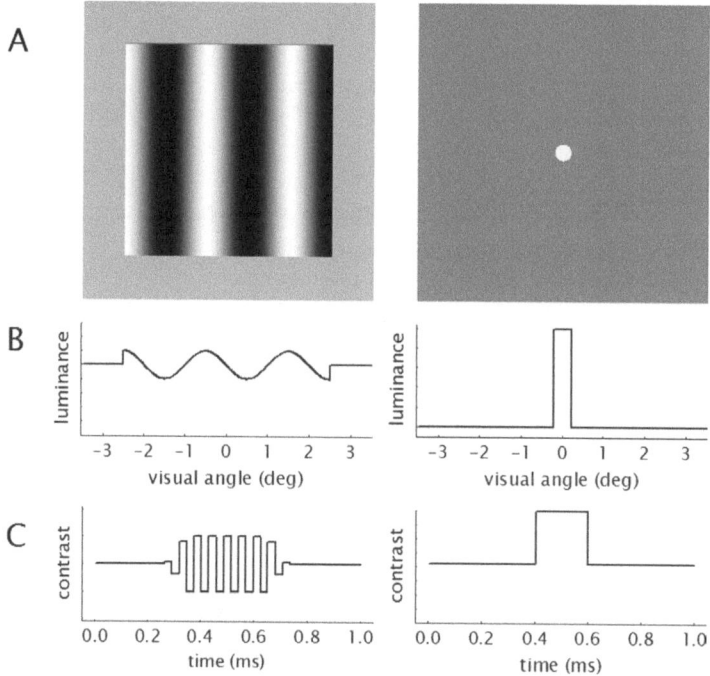

FIGURE 5-1 Visual characteristics of stimuli used in second-generation frequency doubling technology (FDT2) and static automated threshold perimetry (SAP).
NOTES: Compared with stimuli (A) for SAP (right), those for FDT2 (left) display a "flickering" effect in bands across a subsection of the field of vision rather than appearing at a single point (B). The contrast of FDT2 stimuli with the background also flickers over time rather than appearing consistently for a brief span (C).
SOURCE: Artes et al. (2005), reproduced with permission from ARVO.

The FDT perimeter has the capacity to test with both suprathreshold strategies (such as the C-20-1 and C-20-5 patterns in the central 20 degrees) and threshold strategies (such as the N-20 and N-30). A total of 17 points are tested in the C-20 and N-20 programs. When the N-30 program is used, additional points are added nasally. When a threshold program is used, the test may take as long as 4–5 minutes; on the other hand, a suprathreshold test requires less than 1 minute per eye.

Research has demonstrated that the first-generation FDT device performs well in detecting glaucomatous visual field loss (Artes et al., 2005; Cello et al., 2000). The second generation of FDT (FDT2), also known as the FDT Matrix, presents these stimuli on a cathode ray tube with a background luminance of 100 cd/m^2 for 500 milliseconds each (Artes et al., 2005).

The main difference between FDT2 and the first-generation FDT device (FDT1) is the size of the stimuli used. The stimuli in FDT2 are smaller than those used in FDT1, allowing for examination of a larger number of visual field locations (Artes et al., 2005). The result is greater detail on the spatial distribution of visual field loss, allowing greater similarity to the 24-2 and 30-2 patterns used in SAP. Moreover, while FD1 tested only 17–19 locations, FDT2 assesses contrast sensitivity at as many as 54–69 locations (corresponding to 24-2 or 30-2 SAP, respectively). FDT2 uses Bayesian statistical estimation to select stimulus locations based on the examinee's previous responses. This testing strategy has been demonstrated to reduce the variability in testing as well as the duration of testing by 40–50 percent (Shaarawy et al., 2015). Moreover, it is recommended that refractive errors should be corrected prior to testing, since FDT2 devices may cause a loss of optical focus.

This strategy of basing an examinee's threshold using statistical modeling based on their responses is similar to that seen in current versions of SAP. However, in contrast with Humphrey's Swedish Interactive Threshold Algorithm (SITA) algorithm for estimating field loss in SAP, FDT2 presents four stimuli at each location regardless of the level of field loss. This ensures a uniform test duration, whereas SITA ceases to test at locations in the visual field when it determines statistically that an examinee's threshold does not reach that location (Artes et al., 2005).

The results from FDT are typically displayed as a map of the visual field, known as a pattern deviation plot, that highlights areas of normal and abnormal sensitivity. Like the output from SAP, sensitivity (and therefore deviation) is reported in decibels (see Figure 5-2). Clinicians can analyze these data points quantitatively to assess the presence and extent of visual field defects, which can be critical for diagnosing conditions such as glaucoma and monitoring disease progression, thus assisting physicians in clinical decision making.

SPECIAL TOPICS 107

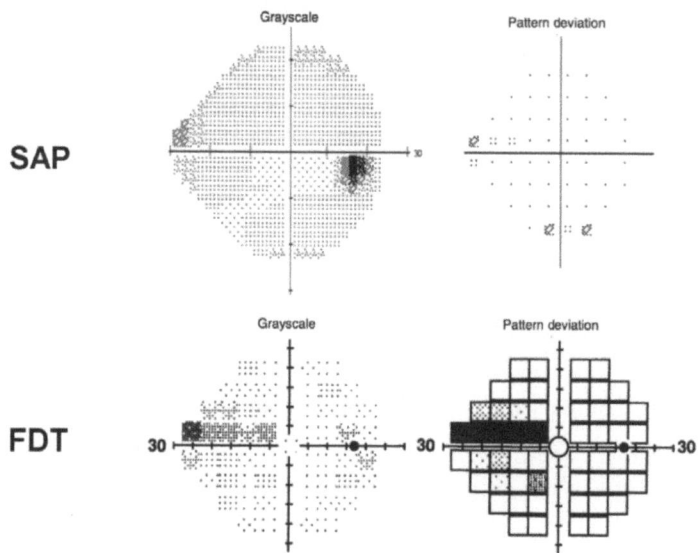

FIGURE 5-2 Visual field from static automated threshold perimetry (SAP) and frequency doubling technology (FDT).
NOTES: The figure presents the visual field from a Humphrey Field Analyzer demonstrating a superior nasal step in the right eye of a patient (SAP) and a representation of the visual field from the FDT device, also showing a superior nasal step. Both visual fields are drawn from early in the disease course of glaucoma.
SOURCE: Tatham et al. (2015). Reprinted with permission from Elsevier.

FDT has several advantages compared with other devices or techniques, such as the Humphrey Field Analyzer and the Octopus. These advantages include the instrument's portability, the ability to perform the test in ambient light, and the added comfort of allowing examinees to wear their own spectacles during testing. FDT also generally requires less training for examiners, and machines using FDT tend to be less expensive. Another advantage of FDT over SAP is that FDT features less response variability along the range of visual field losses it can measure, which makes it particularly useful for monitoring changes in visual field sensitivity over time (Spry et al., 2001). In particular, this explains FDT's effectiveness at detecting early glaucomatous loss, when the differences from a healthy visual field are smaller and less likely to be detected. As a result, FDT features less response variability along the range of visual field losses it can measure; this makes it particularly useful for monitoring changes in visual field sensitivity over time.

The human visual system has different pathways for processing visual information, including the magnocellular (M) and parvocellular (P) pathways. The M-pathway is particularly sensitive to motion and flickering, while the P-pathway is more sensitive to color and fine detail. FDT primarily stimulates the M-pathway, which is thought to be affected more in conditions such as glaucoma. As a result, FDT is often more sensitive to early visual field loss caused by these conditions as compared with traditional perimetry methods. Other approaches can be used for individuals with deficits in the P-pathway.

Because FDT reports sensitivity similarly to traditional perimetry techniques such as SAP, SSA could theoretically use it for disability determination. However, assessing the accuracy and similarity of the results obtained with the two technologies will be important to determining whether such use is feasible.

Comparison of FDT with Traditional Perimeters

The majority of research comparing FDT with standard perimetry has been conducted in the context of detecting early glaucomatous field loss. For early or otherwise mild glaucoma-related visual field loss, studies have shown that FDT performs as well as or better than SAP (Burnstein et al., 2000; Ferreras et al., 2007). FDT has also been shown to display results comparable to those obtained with SAP when used with people who have optic nerve disorders or postchiasmal visual field defects (Huang et al., 2008; Wall et al., 2002; Yoon et al., 2012).

Since people applying for SSA disability benefits will typically have relatively more severe impairments, the relevance of these findings to accuracy in SSA disability determinations is unclear at best. In populations with more severe conditions, comparisons between SAP using the Humphrey Field Analyzer and FDT have yielded mixed results, with some studies showing lower levels of agreement and others showing higher levels of agreement between the two (Artes et al., 2005; Casson and James, 2005; Clement et al., 2009; Doozandeh et al., 2017; Haymes et al., 2005).

Because of its portability and ease of use in the community, FDT has held promise for screening populations. However, some studies suggest that this application of FDT may not be the most effective approach. For example, Boland and colleagues (2016) concluded that FDT, as a stand-alone test, does not have the sensitivity and specificity necessary to detect conditions that may cause serious impairment, such as glaucoma and retinal degeneration, because it likely underestimates the degree of field loss in such examinees. FDT may also not provide sufficiently reliable results in patients with cataracts, making it difficult to determine whether there is a defect using this technology (Casson and James, 2006). On the other hand, there may be some benefits to using FDT with individuals who are inexperienced with perimetric testing (Pierre-Filho Pde et al., 2006).

Conclusions

In summary, FDT is a specialized method that utilizes high-frequency flickering stimuli to assess the integrity of the visual field. It is typically used as a screening test, especially for early or mild visual field impairment caused by glaucoma. Perimeters using FDT tend to be less expensive and easier to use than SAP for both clinicians and examinees.

FDT and SAP tend to display similar results for early or mild glaucomatous impairment. Although findings across studies are mixed regarding FDT's sensitivity, specificity, and agreement with SAP, these differences are greatest in cases of severe impairment. FDT also gives very poor results in patients with cataracts, making it difficult to interpret results and potentially leading to results that may not reflect a true defect. Ultimately, more research validating the use of FDT for diagnostic tasks such as those performed by SSA is needed.

Based on its review of the literature and the committee's expert assessment, the committee reached the following conclusions:

Conclusion 5.3: Second-generation frequency doubling technology (FDT2) devices have demonstrated similarity to traditional perimeters in the measurement of visual field contrast sensitivity; however, most studies thus far have been conducted in individuals with mild to moderate visual impairment. Additional studies are needed to determine the suitability of these devices for assessing visual function in individuals with severe visual impairment.

Conclusion 5.4: Because of its portability and lower cost, frequency doubling technology is likely to be particularly useful in settings where patients have limited access to static automated threshold perimetry and other traditional perimeters.

SEMIAUTOMATED KINETIC PERIMETRY[3]

As discussed in Chapter 3, the stimulus presented in a perimetry test can be either *static* or *kinetic*. In static perimetry, stimuli are presented one at a time at defined points in the visual field, and examinees are asked to indicate when they see a stimulus. Stimuli presented for longer durations of time may be seen better as a result of temporal summation of information,

---

[3] In much of the literature, as well as in the SSA listings and in this report's statement of task, the term *automated kinetic perimetry* is commonly used as interchangeable with *semiautomated kinetic perimetry*. However, this report uses the term *semiautomated kinetic perimetry* to make clear the role of the examiner in performing this type of examination.

although limited additional benefit is derived beyond times over 0.1 second. Most commonly used static perimeters, such as the Humphrey Field Analyzer and the Octopus, are automated. Before the test, the examiner typically selects the size of the stimulus, and then the visual field test is executed using the instrument's software and algorithm. Static perimeters are widely available, relatively fast, and particularly sensitive to detecting early visual field loss from glaucoma. Compared with kinetic perimeters, however, they require greater patient concentration and may be less efficient in delineating complex lesions that extend into the peripheral field and localizing occipital lobe lesions.

In kinetic perimetry, the stimulus is usually moved from an area without vision ("subthreshold") to one with vision ("suprathreshold"), and the examiner records the location at which the stimulus is first seen. To test different areas of the visual field, this process is repeated along multiple meridians (i.e., differently angled lines through the center of the visual field). The speed at which the stimulus is moved should be standardized and typically ranges from 2 to 4 degrees per second. This technique tests the thresholds of a person's visual field directly.

The stimulus can also be moved from a seeing area to a nonseeing area, which may be especially helpful in mapping out more complex ring scotomas. Employing both methods may minimize the bias in outlining intricate islands of vision, such as those associated with conditions such as retinitis pigmentosa. Testing in both directions can therefore provide useful clinical information in some cases.

Even so, it is relatively uncommon; losing out on this information (such as by only performing the typical method of kinetic perimetry) is unlikely to affect Social Security disability benefits eligibility for the vast majority of applicants. Since the measurement of disability requires estimating the extent of the visual field along standardized meridians, the usual subthreshold-to-suprathreshold method is unlikely to underestimate visual field loss as it relates to disability, except for people with central visual loss, such as might be seen with macular degeneration, and those people often have disabling levels of visual acuity or would qualify for disability benefits otherwise.

Unlike static perimeters, most kinetic perimetry techniques, including Goldmann perimetry and tangent screening (detailed in Chapter 2), are manual; that is, the examiner physically moves the stimulus and records the examinee's responses. This makes the test relatively time consuming, and the manual element creates a risk of bias and nonreproducibility in the results (Bevers et al., 2019). However, a skilled examiner can assess the likelihood of error during the test based on the plausibility of reported results (Mönter et al., 2017). This capability can mitigate the possible response bias introduced by single self-reported responses close to a threshold.

Fully automated, computer-guided kinetic perimetry may theoretically eliminate examiner bias, but it would not be able to mitigate response bias. Moreover, preset automated kinetic testing patterns, such as those available for the Humphrey Field Analyzer, may not offer the flexibility to search for more central scotomas. As a result, fully automated kinetic perimetry has not been widely validated in the literature, nor is it widely available (Bevers et al., 2019; Mönter et al., 2017).

Semiautomated kinetic perimetry is more common. In this method, the examiner still sets the size and intensity of the stimulus, while the pattern and movement of stimuli are controlled by a computer. This method combines automated features with manual retest and customized testing patterns to allow for greater flexibility. The speed and test pattern are standardized, and greater accuracy in examinee responses is achieved (Barnes et al., 2019). By comparing the advantages and disadvantages conferred by this type of automation with manual methods, SSA can consider the additional value that semiautomated kinetic perimetry can bring to disability determinations.

Kinetic Perimetry for Social Security Disability Determinations

For SSA disability determination, manual or semiautomated kinetic perimetry is used primarily for assessing visual field efficiency pursuant to Section 2.03C of the listings. Under this section, SSA calculates a person's "visual field efficiency," which corresponds to the percentage of a typical visual field that a person can see through their better eye. Specifically, visual field efficiency is calculated by adding the number of degrees a patient sees along the eight "principal" meridians found on a visual field chart (Figure 5-3), each located 45 degrees apart, in their better eye, and dividing by five. Since the extent of the normal visual field at each meridian adds up to 500,[4] the sum of the patient's extent along each meridian is divided by five to calculate their visual field efficiency. To meet the minimum listing criteria for disability in Section 2.03C, the visual field efficiency in the better eye must be 20 percent or less after this calculation. A more detailed discussion of SSA's methodology can be found in Chapter 1.

---

[4] SSA's normal visual field extent at the eight principal meridians is 85 degrees (temporally), 60 degrees (up temporally), 45 degrees (superiorly), 55 degrees (up nasally), 60 degrees (nasally), 55 degrees (down nasally), 60 degrees (inferiorly), and 80 degrees (down temporally) (SSA, n.d., 2.00A7cB).

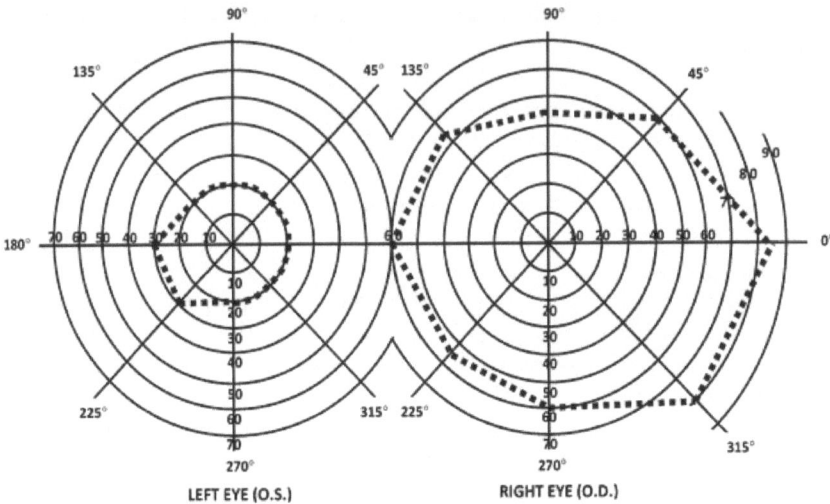

FIGURE 5-3 Diagram of the eight principal meridians for each eye.
NOTE: The diagram for the right eye shows a typical visual field extent drawn in dashed lines. The diagram for the left eye shows a constrained visual field; a healthy visual field would be a mirror image of the right eye's field shape. In addition, the degrees assigned to each meridian are *not* mirrored and instead remain the same.
SOURCE: SSA (n.d., 2.00A7cB).

Validity and Reliability of Semiautomated Kinetic Perimetry

Results obtained with semiautomated kinetic perimetry are similar to those obtained with typical manual kinetic perimetry. Differences found in the literature between visual fields measured with semiautomated and manual kinetic methods are generally either small or not statistically significant (Barnes et al., 2019; Hashimoto et al., 2017; Nowomiejska et al., 2005; Rowe and Rowlands, 2014). The two types of kinetic perimetry have similar test durations (Patel et al., 2018; Rowe and Rowlands, 2014).

More important, however, is the ability of semiautomated kinetic perimetry to yield results similar to those obtained with the "gold standard" Humphrey Field Analyzer and other static automated threshold perimeters. If the outputs are similar, then SSA's assessment of disability is likely to be similar using either technique. As discussed in Chapter 4, studies comparing disability evaluation findings using each method would have been the most informative for this report; however, the committee found no such studies in the literature. Direct comparisons of field size or radius found via static and kinetic perimetry are similarly difficult because of mathematical differences in the respective methodologies

(Christofofridis, 2011). Therefore, comparisons between semiautomated kinetic perimetry and SAP tend to focus on diagnostic agreement, test duration, and test–retest reliability.

It is important to note that diagnostic agreement between semiautomated kinetic perimetry and SAP may be condition dependent. Studies assessing diagnostic agreement compare perimeters across several measures, such as match rate of visual field identification as normal or abnormal, defect type, and defect severity. Table 5-2 summarizes such studies comparing semiautomated kinetic perimetry from an Octopus perimeter with SAP from a Humphrey Field Analyzer.

TABLE 5-2 Diagnostic Agreement Between Octopus Semiautomated Kinetic Perimetry and Humphrey Field Analyzer Static Automated Perimetry

Study	Year	N	Clinical Context	Metric	% Agreement	Notes
Rowe et al.	2013	64 patients, 113 eyes	Neuro-ophthalmic disease	Normal/abnormal	73.5%	I4e target
				Normal/abnormal	80%	I2e target
				Normal/abnormal	87%	Combined
Nowomiejska et al.	2009	13 patients, 26 eyes	Bilateral visible optic nerve head drusen	Clinical description	73%	
Bhaskaran et al.	2021	17 patients, 26 eyes	Various	Normal/abnormal	88%	
				Normal/abnormal	80%–89%	By quadrant
				Diagnostic pattern	54%–65%	
				Diagnostic pattern	95%	Central and paracentral scotomata excluded
Rowe et al.	2015	50 patients, 100 eyes	Pituitary disease	Defect type	58%	
				Defect severity	50%	
Patel et al.	2019	30 patients, 60 eyes	Pediatric neuro-ophthalmic disease	Defect type	69%	
				Defect severity	50%	

The agreement found in the literature between these two types of perimeters ranges from moderate to good. Semiautomated kinetic perimetry demonstrates a good ability to differentiate between normal and abnormal visual fields as compared with the same identification performed with SAP (Bhaskaran et al., 2021; Rowe et al., 2013). However, results are less similar when clinical features such as defect type and severity are matched (Bhaskaran et al., 2021; Nowomiejska et al., 2009; Patel et al., 2015; Rowe et al., 2015).

It is important to note that while semiautomated kinetic perimetry tests along an entire meridian and can test the full visual field, static perimetry of all types samples individual points in the visual field and typically tests only the central portion of the field. Some of the differences in agreement between the techniques may be due to the differences in how each technique measures the visual field rather than potential weaknesses in a technique's ability to perform such measurement.

Bhaskaran and colleagues (2021), however, found that once readings featuring central and paracentral scotomatas were excluded, the sensitivity of the Octopus (semiautomated kinetic) perimeter for detecting defects increased to 95 percent when the Humphrey Field Analyzer (static automated threshold perimeter) was used as a baseline. This finding is consistent with findings that semiautomated kinetic perimetry performs best at assessing the peripheral visual field, findings that are also reflected in SSA's preference for manual kinetic perimetry or SAP when scotomatas or other severe constrictions in the central visual field are indicated. Weaknesses of SAP in measuring visual field loss at the periphery, as well as their implications for measuring against the SSA criteria, are discussed in a later section.

With respect to differences in test duration between static and kinetic methods, evidence is mixed as well (Nowomiejska et al., 2015; Rowe et al., 2013, 2015, 2021).

Finally, the test–retest reliability of semiautomated kinetic perimetry is similar to that of SAP (Mönter et al., 2017; Nevalainen et al., 2008).

In general, despite some findings of only moderate agreement, kinetic perimetry offers several unique advantages over static perimetry, many of which have been specifically demonstrated in semiautomated kinetic perimetry. For example, because static perimetry typically tests only the central visual field, it may fail to detect "residual islands of sensitivity" in the mid-periphery or periphery (Patel et al., 2018). This may occur with conditions such as retinitis pigmentosa or other retinal dystrophies commonly needing disability determination. On the other hand, because kinetic perimetry can test the full field of vision, it is preferred for testing the peripheral visual field (Keltner et al., 1999; Simpson, 2017). Semiautomated kinetic perimetry also can supplement static perimetry when additional information about the periphery would be clinically useful (Ma et al., 2021; Patel et al., 2018; Rowe et al., 2021). Kinetic perimetry may also be preferred for examining visual fields in children. Even though semiautomated kinetic perimetry can entail longer test durations in a pediatric setting, they tend to be more feasible for children compared with SAP (Patel et al., 2015; Wilscher et al., 2010).

However, the primary advantage of semiautomated kinetic perimetry is its ability to standardize the movement of a stimulus. In manual kinetic perimetry, the examiner moves the stimulus, which leads to considerable interoperator variability in stimulus velocity and examiner reaction time. While patient reaction time remains a factor in both semiautomated and manual kinetic perimetry, examiner biases can be reduced with semiautomated methods (Bhaskaran et al., 2021; Nowomiejska et al., 2010). Further standardization of measurement procedures has eliminated differential results between semiautomated kinetic perimetry and SAP in some studies (Phu et al., 2016, 2018).

Conclusion

Semiautomated kinetic perimetry can be used to determine disability as defined by SSA. It can be used to evaluate peripheral defects outside the central 30 degrees of the visual field (i.e., to the full 90 degrees with a range of 47 dB), a requirement for calculating visual field efficiency as defined by SSA (Section 2.03C). Regarding other pathways to qualifying for disability benefits, semiautomated kinetic perimetry adds value over manual kinetic perimetry because the learning curve is shorter, and operators require less technical expertise and training.

At the same time, however, kinetic perimetry (either manual or semiautomated) has limitations. It tends to be less concordant with static methods when the central visual field is being assessed and, therefore, is often suggested in the literature to be used at the periphery (Mönter et al., 2017; Rowe et al., 2015). To realize the full potential of kinetic perimetry for full-field and peripheral visual field assessment, an examiner needs experience and training beyond that required by static perimetry. A skilled technician can monitor for fixation loss, check for false negatives or positives, and plot more complicated scotomas. In particular, ineffective monitoring of fixation can lead to overestimation of visual field performance. As a result, static perimetry may be preferred if there is generalized constriction of the visual field, and neither peripheral "islands of vision" nor ring scotomas are likely. SAP uses standardized algorithms to plot threshold sensitivities within the central 48–60 degrees of the visual field automatically.

Acquiring an Octopus perimeter (the most common platform capable of performing semiautomated kinetic testing) may be prohibitively expensive, and even where these perimeters are available, adequately trained technicians may not be available outside specialized clinics. If Octopus perimeters were the only machines SSA considered acceptable for employing semiautomated kinetic strategies, then given the associated cost and training constraints, permitting the use of semiautomated kinetic perimetry could lead to only modest improvements in the availability of visual field testing. On the other hand, some clinics may have only an Octopus or other semiautomated kinetic perimeter, or an individual clinician may prefer using semiautomated kinetic perimetry.

Based on its review of the literature, the committee reached the following conclusion:

Conclusion 5.5: When administered by a skilled technician, semiautomated kinetic perimetry has sufficient accuracy in quantifying visual field efficiency for use by SSA in disability determinations.

ALTERNATIVES TO KINETIC PERIMETRY FOR TESTING VISUAL FIELD EFFICIENCY

As discussed above and in Chapter 1, the SSA listings allow for a determination of disability with the finding of a visual field efficiency of less than or equal to 20 percent in the better eye after SSA's calculation in Section 2.03C is applied. Manual kinetic perimetry (most commonly performed with a Goldmann perimeter) and semiautomated kinetic perimetry (most commonly performed with an Octopus perimeter) are the two types of tests SSA permits for measurement of visual field efficiency. Other tests, including SAP and those considered to be screening methods, such as confrontation tests or tangent screens, are not currently permitted for measurement of visual field efficiency.

Results from SAP could theoretically be used to calculate visual field efficiency. An examiner could use a transparent overlay outlining the eight principal meridians on the results (or printout) from a Humphrey Field Analyzer or similar static automated threshold perimeter to calculate the visual field limits as required under Section 2.03C. This approach would be in line with disability determination procedures of other agencies (see Chapter 2), which allow for the use of other methods, including SAP.

These automated static methods can consist of either threshold tests, which calculate the precise sensitivity of various locations in the eye, or suprathreshold tests, which instead make a binary determination as to whether a stimulus is visible at the same locations. While SSA typically uses threshold testing, such as most perimetry performed using a Humphrey Field Analyzer, an alternative could be the use of tests that display suprathreshold stimuli (i.e., stimuli that are significantly brighter than the expected threshold of visual detection) at every test location. The goal of this testing would not be to determine the precise sensitivity at any specific spot in the visual field but would be to make a simple binary determination as to whether an examinee could see at that location. As a result, suprathreshold tests are typically used as screening tests.

Utility of Screening Tests in SSA Disability Determination

Screening tests usually take less time than threshold tests. Furthermore, they can measure the periphery farther out than is possible with threshold tests. In addition, screening tests can be performed with both eyes to evaluate for binocular field loss, such as might be seen from postchiasmatic (i.e., farther down the optic nerve) damage to the visual pathways. Indeed, a recent survey of neuro-ophthalmologists indicated that the Esterman (monocular and binocular) and 120-point screening strategies were on the "short list" of preferred methods for evaluating the visual sequelae of common conditions such as stroke, optic neuropathy, and chiasmic compression (Hepworth and Rowe, 2019).

Since screening tests employ suprathreshold brightness, they may underestimate the full extent of visual field loss (i.e., have lower sensitivity) compared with a threshold test (Ayala, 2012). In the appropriate clinical setting, a screening test demonstrating sufficient visual field loss for a determination of disability under SSA policy would not require further testing with a threshold test. However, a patient with suspected or known visual field loss whose screening test did not demonstrate sufficient field loss to support a disability claim might require further testing with a threshold strategy. In summary, screening methods may yield reliable results depending on the details of the screening method and the examinee's circumstances.

Differences between Static and Kinetic Perimetry Relevant to Disability Determination

A detailed comparison of the use of static and kinetic perimetry for visual field assessment and disability determination can be found in the prior section. When multiple methods are permitted for disability evaluation, it is important that they either yield similar results in similar circumstances or have distinct advantages in evaluating different clinical presentations. In either case, all acceptable methods would ideally qualify and disqualify the same people for SSA disability benefits. However, static perimetry faces two methodological challenges as a potential alternative to kinetic perimetry for measurement of visual field efficiency: First, as noted earlier, static perimetry used in the clinical setting typically measures only the central 60 degrees of the visual field. Second, SSA requires that static perimetry tests use the size III Goldmann stimulus.

Peripheral Visual Field Measurement

As discussed in the previous section, SSA defines visual field efficiency as the sum of the extent of a person's visual field across each of eight principal meridians divided by five. In other words, it is the percentage of a typical visual field that a person can see through their better eye. Calculating visual field efficiency requires an assessment of the full visual field, since vision along some meridians typically extends out to 85 degrees from the point of central fixation.

Current algorithms for visual field threshold estimation, such as the SITA available on Humphrey and Octopus perimeters, generally do not support measurement at the outer peripheral fields. Examiners can use these algorithms for peripheral threshold testing, but the mathematical models are not as well validated for the periphery. The result is longer testing times, even with ideal testing methodology for the far periphery (Wall et al., 2019). Test duration, in turn, is inversely related to reliability (Yohannan et al., 2017). As a result, many automated static perimeters provide test patterns that do not extend to the farthest reaches of the periphery. However, they may be still labeled as "full field" patterns. Examples include the following:

- The Humphrey Field Analyzer's 60-4 test measures 60 points from 30 to 60 degrees (Carl Zeiss Meditec, 2003).
- The Octopus perimeter's N pattern measures 71 points extending from 40 degrees nasally to 67 degrees temporally and 40 degrees vertically (Racette et al., 2019).
- The Octopus perimeter's 07 pattern measures 130 points extending from 70 degrees temporally to 55 degrees nasally (Racette et al., 2019).

Notably, these strategies do not fully contain all the points required by SSA for the calculation of visual field efficiency.

Stimulus Size

SSA currently requires that SAP tests use a white size III Goldmann stimulus, which is 0.43 degrees in diameter and 4 mm^2 in area. Although no type of static perimetry is currently allowed for the measurement of visual field efficiency (it is used primarily in other methods for visual field–based disability evaluation), the requirement for a size III stimulus would make such assessments difficult if they were allowed.

Most static perimeters can also use a Goldmann size V stimulus, which is 1.72 degrees in diameter and 64 mm^2 in area. Size V stimuli are used most commonly to test people with extremely low vision (Morgan et al., 2019). However, when used for routine perimetric testing and monitoring of people with various visual impairments, size V stimuli have been found to maintain several advantages over size III stimuli.

Because size V stimuli are larger, they are easier to notice when all else is held equal. Since the examinee is able to respond to more stimuli, using a size V stimulus increases test duration (Sood et al., 2021). Typically, a longer test duration reduces reliability (Yohannan et al., 2017). However, studies of perimetry using size V stimuli consistently report lower test–retest variability and higher repeatability (Davis et al., 2011; Flanagan et al., 2016; Gardiner et al., 2013; Wall et al., 2008, 2013). This is likely because using a size V stimulus increases sensitivity; a person who has sight in a part of their visual field is more likely to notice a larger stimulus than a smaller one (Gardiner et al., 2013; Morgan et al., 2019).

In theory, larger stimuli may be more apparent to people with early impairment. For example, larger stimuli could stimulate the healthy, seeing regions surrounding a scotoma (Gardiner et al., 2015). However, several studies have found no significant difference between size III stimuli and size V stimuli in the number of points detected (Flanagan et al., 2016; Phu et al., 2017; Wall et al., 2013). When stratifying by the examinee's mean deviation (i.e., average sensitivity deviation from normal values for all measured visual field locations), Wall and colleagues (2013) found that size V stimuli were the most sensitive. While these larger stimuli may result in slightly different mean deviation scores, the committee believes that this difference will not impact determination outcomes for most people with severe enough defects to be evaluated by SSA. Moreover, when size V stimuli are used because of a person's poor visual acuity, that visual acuity may qualify them for disability benefits anyway. As a result, reliability for the classification task considered in this report is unlikely to be affected by underestimations of defect depth.

Larger stimuli may perform better in particular at the far periphery. Flanagan and colleagues (2016) found that a size V stimulus was detectable at more locations outside the central visual field, a finding consistent with findings that outside of the central 30 degrees from the point of central fixation, size III stimuli have worse variability and sensitivity (Wall et al., 2019). Given that measurement of visual field efficiency requires assessment of the full visual field, use of a size V stimulus would likely result in more reliable results for disability determination purposes.

Conclusion

While SAP is available to measure peripheral vision, it may not suffice for measuring the full extent of the visual field as required by SSA for the calculation of visual field efficiency. For most people seeking disability benefits, however, this limitation does not make much of a difference; a person found to qualify for disability benefits using a 60 degree perimeter likely would have a sufficiently constrained visual field to qualify, and would not need additional testing with a perimeter to test further boundaries. Furthermore, SAP is far more commonly available today than semiautomated kinetic perimetry, and it can be performed with more consistency and less examiner bias than manual kinetic perimetry.

Allowing the use of static automated threshold perimetry for assessing visual field efficiency may yield uncertain or inadequate results in some scenarios. Since all of the current commercially available instruments and testing methods have their own limitations with respect to the clinical information they provide, multiple tests with the same method or an array of methods may be required to provide a better understanding of the extent of visual field loss. For example, kinetic perimetry could be used to determine the extent of the peripheral visual field, while a more centrally focused SAP test could be used to establish the extent of the central field.

Although SAP is not a "one-to-one" substitution for manual or semiautomated kinetic perimetry, it usually can provide the data required to calculate visual field efficiency. However, there may be rare exceptions. It is theoretically possible that a ring scotoma, such as those seen in retinitis pigmentosa, could leave the entire visual field past 60 degrees unaffected. Using SAP for visual field efficiency measurement could result in a technical "false positive" that would result in approving that person for disability benefits. However, the committee believes that the overall disability experienced by such a patient with significant ring scotomas or midperipheral visual field loss is otherwise likely to provide sufficient evidence to result in a disability determination.

Use of a larger stimulus size can increase the reliability of SAP at the periphery. The currently mandated size III Goldmann stimulus has resulted in increased intertest variability and lower sensitivity, especially at the periphery. Size III stimuli may be sufficient for testing the central visual field, and therefore sufficient for disability determinations not based on visual field efficiency. However, a size V stimulus would be more feasible and reliable if SAP were used to assess visual field efficiency.

Based on its review of the literature, the committee reached the following conclusions:

Conclusion 5.6: Despite the limitations of static automated threshold perimetry (SAP) in measuring peripheral field loss, this method can usually provide the data necessary to calculate the visual field efficiency of an applicant for SSA disability benefits.

- *Visual field efficiencies calculated using SAP will generally be diagnostically equivalent to those calculated using currently approved manual (Goldmann) kinetic or semiautomated kinetic*

perimetry; applicants who qualify for benefits using one will almost always qualify using the other.
- Even in exceedingly rare scenarios in which a person qualifies for disability benefits based on SAP assessment of visual field efficiency whereas in fact, the regions of the peripheral visual field outside the region mapped by SAP have preserved vision to a degree that the true visual field efficiency would not meet SSA requirements, the overall disability experienced by the applicant is likely to provide sufficient evidence to result in a disability determination.

Conclusion 5.7: The use of larger stimuli, further diagnostic tests, and other clinical data can improve the diagnostic reliability of static automated threshold perimetry for the calculation of visual field efficiency.

PEDIATRIC CONSIDERATIONS

Childhood visual disability is a significant public health concern in the United States. The number of pediatric ophthalmologists is limited nationally, and access to pediatric eye care is particularly poor in rural and other medically underserved areas (Oatts et al., 2023; Walsh et al., 2023). Lack of access to timely vision screenings or eye care can lead to unnecessary vision loss; approximately half of all childhood blindness is preventable or treatable (Lim et al., 2023).

In the present context, obtaining diagnoses and information necessary to meet SSA's disability criteria may also be delayed. These diagnoses are already challenging; perimetry has several limitations when performed in children, which can further exacerbate their difficulties in receiving disability benefits for visual field loss.

Equipment Challenges in Pediatric Perimetry

Device-specific considerations relevant to children include physical discomfort; lack of age-specific normative databases; and the role of emerging technology, such as VR perimetry.

Standard perimetry hardware, such as the Humphrey Field Analyzer, was developed for adults, which makes positioning a child for perimetry difficult. Often, for example, children's feet cannot reach the ground. This physical discomfort can have a negative influence on test reliability. As mentioned previously, VR perimetry is an emerging technology that holds significant promise for use in children for this reason. VR devices eliminate the ergonomic concerns related to larger, traditional perimeters. Children can sit or stand comfortably, although very young children may find the VR headset heavy or too large. VR perimetry may also appeal to children because of its novelty and similarity to other technologies they enjoy, such as screen- and VR-based games. Child-specific algorithms, such as those asking examinees to land a rocket spaceship on a planet, can incorporate elements of game playing and keep the child engaged during testing (Groth et al., 2023).

The literature evaluating the use of VR perimetry in children is nascent but growing (Groth et al., 2023; Mesfin et al., 2024; Wang et al., 2023). Generally, these studies have shown good correlation with traditional perimetry, as well as high levels of acceptability in children. The same limitations of these devices in adults—the validity of screen-based stimuli and the presence or absence of eye-tracking technology to ensure fixation—apply also to children.

Statistical Challenges in Pediatric Perimetry

Another limitation entailed in interpreting the results of perimetry in children is the absence of comprehensive normative databases specifically for this population. Such databases offer a statistical profile of a typical population with regard to visual field extent. Automated static perimeters, such as the Humphrey Field Analyzer, use these databases as part of their mathematical modeling of the examinee's visual field.

Adult normative databases may not be directly applicable to younger populations. Several independent research groups have worked to publish normative databases for children using both standard and emerging technologies (Groth et al., 2023; Patel et al., 2015). While these efforts are important, they may not readily or automatically be integrated into the test printouts from device manufacturers. Until the typical visual field extents for children are better understood and normative databases have been published, however, greater methodological flexibility may make it easier for children with visual field loss to access disability benefits.

The reliability of visual field tests is a special consideration in children as well. Younger children may not be able to complete a visual field test because of lack of understanding or cooperation, and children who do complete the testing may produce unreliable results based on traditional reliability metrics. A study of more than 100 children aged 18 and younger with glaucoma or suspected glaucoma found that only approximately half of their visual field tests were considered reliable in this population based on manufacturer-recommended reliability guidelines (Kumar et al., 2024).

Additionally, a significant learning effect was not observed, meaning that children whose first visual field test was unreliable were unlikely to produce reliable tests on subsequent examinations. Factors associated with greater odds of test reliability included older age, better best-corrected visual acuity, and speaking English as the primary language. Finally, the setting for visual field testing can impact results in children. Creating a child-friendly environment can improve test performance, as can the presence of a skilled technician familiar with pediatric patients. These skilled technicians can also offer insight as to a child's visual status, especially when the child is unable to comply with perimetric testing.

Conclusion

Given the practical considerations involved in evaluating visual fields in children across a range of ages and developmental statuses, there is particular value in providing increased flexibility in perimetry requirements in this population. Additionally, newer technologies have the potential to address challenges associated with performing perimetric examinations in children. For example, VR-based platforms may be more comfortable for children than larger traditional perimeters, and they can incorporate design features, such as game-like features and eye tracking, that can keep the child engaged during the test. Saccadic vector optokinetic perimetry, based on principles of oculokinetic perimetry (see Chapter 3), is another option for measuring visual fields in pediatric patients, especially younger children who are not yet able to perform quantitative visual field testing.

In contrast to adults with visual impairment, many children with visual impairment severe enough to qualify for SSA disability benefits have other comorbid health conditions (Salt and Sargent, 2014). In evaluating perimetry to determine visual disability in children, flexibility is needed in the requirement for formal visual field testing in those children who cannot comply with this requirement because of their developmental or health status.

Based on its review of the literature, the committee reached the following conclusion:

Conclusion 5.8: There is particular value in increased flexibility in perimetry requirements for children, given the practical considerations involved in evaluating visual field in this population across a range of ages and developmental and health statuses. Newer technologies, such as screen-based perimeters using perimetry methods that incorporate game-like features or oculokinetic perimetry, have the potential to address these challenges in pediatric perimetry and yield valid information for the identification of SSA-qualifying visual field loss.

SUMMARY

In considering expansion of the perimetric devices allowed as part of SSA's disability determinations, the primary factors to balance are the accessibility of tests and equipment currently required and the ability of a new technique to assess visual field loss accurately, as compared with current methods. While it is important that all approved methods yield results as similar to one another as possible, even the "gold standard" Humphrey Field Analyzer displays intertest variation and sensitivity concerns in certain clinical contexts. While SAP (for visual field efficiency measurement) and frequency doubling technology (for general perimetric use) may not have full concordance with the methods currently preferred by SSA, they are far more available and less expensive, and evidence suggests that they yield measurements similar to those of the currently preferred perimeters. If an individual visual field test does not provide enough information, SSA can request further tests to confirm borderline results. Allowing these alternative techniques would help more people acquire the medical information they need to apply for SSA disability benefits.

Other technologies remain promising but currently lack the evidence base needed to determine their diagnostic agreement with standard methods. In theory, stimuli displayed on LCD and OLED displays can be modified for functional equivalence with Goldmann size III stimuli, but validation studies into screen-based perimetry are nascent. Of particular interest is that emerging technologies such as VR and other screen-based methods can be adapted for use in the pediatric setting. As child-specific perimeters are developed using these platforms, more data will be available to determine their acceptability for disability determination.

REFERENCES

Ahmed, Y., A. Pereira, S. Bowden, R. B. Shi, Y. Li, I. I. K. Ahmed, and S. A. Arshinoff. 2022. Multicenter comparison of the Toronto portable perimeter with the Humphrey field analyzer: A pilot study. *Ophthalmology Glaucoma* 5(2):146–159.

Artes, P. H., D. M. Hutchison, M. T. Nicolela, R. P. LeBlanc, and B. C. Chauhan. 2005. Threshold and variability properties of matrix frequency-doubling technology and standard automated perimetry in glaucoma. *Investigative Ophthalmology & Visual Science* 46(7):2451–2457.

Ayala, M. 2012. Comparison of the monocular Humphrey visual field and the binocular Humphrey Esterman visual field test for driver licensing in glaucoma subjects in Sweden. *BMC Ophthalmology* 12:1–7.

Barnes, C. S., R. A. Schuchard, D. G. Birch, G. Dagnelie, L. Wood, R. K. Koenekoop, and A. K. Bittner. 2019. Reliability of semiautomated kinetic perimetry (SKP) and Goldmann kinetic perimetry in children and adults with retinal dystrophies. *Translational Vision Science & Technology* 8(3):36–36.

Berneshawi, A. R., A. Shue, and R. T. Chang. 2024. Glaucoma home self-testing using VR visual fields and rebound tonometry versus in-clinic perimetry and Goldmann applanation tonometry: A pilot study. *Translational Vision Science & Technology* 13(8):7–7.

Bevers, C., G. Blanckaert, K. Van Keer, J. F. Fils, E. Vandewalle, and I. Stalmans. 2019. Semi-automated kinetic perimetry: Comparison of the Octopus 900 and Humphrey visual field analyzer 3 versus Goldmann perimetry. *Acta Ophthalmologica* 97(4):e499–e505.

Bhaskaran, K., S. Phuljhele, P. Kumar, R. Saxena, D. Angmo, and P. Sharma. 2021. Comparative evaluation of octopus semi-automated kinetic perimeter with Humphrey and Goldmann perimeters in neuro-ophthalmic disorders. *Indian Journal of Ophthalmology* 69(4):918–922.

Boland, M. V., P. Gupta, F. Ko, D. Zhao, E. Guallar, and D. S. Friedman. 2016. Evaluation of frequency-doubling technology perimetry as a means of screening for glaucoma and other eye diseases using the national health and nutrition examination survey. *JAMA Ophthalmology* 134(1):57–62.

Bradley, C., I. I. K. Ahmed, T. W. Samuelson, M. Chaglasian, H. Barnebey, N. Radcliffe, and J. Bacharach. 2024. Validation of a wearable virtual reality perimeter for glaucoma staging, the nova trial: Novel virtual reality field assessment. *Translational Vision Science & Technology* 13(3):10.

Burnstein, Y., N. J. Ellish, M. Magbalon, and E. J. Higginbotham. 2000. Comparison of frequency doubling perimetry with Humphrey visual field analysis in a glaucoma practice. *American Journal of Ophthalmology* 129(3):328–333.

Carl Zeiss Meditec. 2003. *Humphrey Field Analyzer II - i Series User's Guide*. https://acmerevival.com/wp-content/uploads/2021/05/Zeiss-Humphrey-HFA-II-720i-Visual-Field-AnalyzerUserManual.pdf (accessed February 3, 2025).

Casson, R. J., and B. James. 2006. Effect of cataract on frequency doubling perimetry in the screening mode. *Journal of Glaucoma* 15(1):23–25.

Cello, K. E., J. M. Nelson-Quigg, and C. A. Johnson. 2000. Frequency doubling technology perimetry for detection of glaucomatous visual field loss. *American Journal of Ophthalmology* 129(3):314–322.

Chia, Z. K., A. W. Kong, M. L. Turner, M. Saifee, B. E. Damato, B. T. Backus, J. J. Blaha, J. S. Schuman, M. S. Deiner, and Y. Ou. 2024. Assessment of remote training, at-home testing, and test-retest variability of a novel test for clustered virtual reality perimetry. *Ophthalmology Glaucoma* 7(2):139–147.

Christoforidis, J. B. 2011. Volume of visual field assessed with kinetic perimetry and its application to static perimetry. *Clinical Ophthalmology* 5:535–541.

Clement, C. I., I. Goldberg, P. R. Healey, and S. Graham. 2009. Humphrey matrix frequency doubling perimetry for detection of visual-field defects in open-angle glaucoma. *The British Journal of Ophthalmology* 93(5):582–588.

Davis, C. E., C. K. Doyle, G. J. Zamba, C. A. Johnson, and M. Wall. 2011. The effect of stimulus size on repeatability in glaucoma using Goldmann sizes III, V, VI and STP. *Investigative Ophthalmology & Visual Science* 52(14):5508–5508.

Doozandeh, A., F. Irandoost, A. Mirzajani, S. Yazdani, M. Pakravan, and H. Esfandiari. 2017. Comparison of matrix frequency-doubling technology (FDT) perimetry with the Swedish interactive thresholding algorithm (SIYA) standard automated perimetry (SAP) in mild glaucoma. *Medical Hypothesis, Discovery and Innovation in Ophthalmology* 6(3):98.

Ferreras, A., V. Polo, J. M. Larrosa, L. E. Pablo, A. B. Pajarin, V. Pueyo, and F. M. Honrubia. 2007. Can frequency-doubling technology and short-wavelength automated perimetries detect visual field defects before standard automated perimetry in patients with preperimetric glaucoma? *Journal of Glaucoma* 16(4):372–383.

Flanagan, J. G., P. H. Artes, M. Wall, E. Young, T. Callan, V. M. Patella, M. Monhart, and G. C. Lee. 2016. The influence of perimetric stimulus size on defect detectability in early glaucoma. *Investigative Ophthalmology & Visual Science* 57(12).

Gardiner, S., D. Goren, C. Goldman, W. Swanson, and S. Demirel. 2013. The effect of stimulus size on the relation between sensitivity and variability in perimetry. *Investigative Ophthalmology & Visual Science* 54(15):2636–2636.

Gardiner, S. K., S. Demirel, D. Goren, S. L. Mansberger, and W. H. Swanson. 2015. The effect of stimulus size on the reliable stimulus range of perimetry. *Translational Vision Science & Technology* 4(2):10.

Grau, E., S. Andrae, F. Horn, B. Hohberger, M. Ring, and G. Michelson. 2023. Teleglaucoma using a new smartphone-based tool for visual field assessment. *Journal of Glaucoma* 32(3):186–194.

Greenfield, J. A., M. Deiner, A. Nguyen, G. Wollstein, B. Damato, B. T. Backus, M. Wu, J. S. Schuman, and Y. Ou. 2022. Virtual reality oculokinetic perimetry test reproducibility and relationship to conventional perimetry and OCT. *Ophthalmology Science* 2(1):100105.

Grobbel, J., J. Dietzsch, C. A. Johnson, R. Vonthein, K. Stingl, R. G. Weleber, and U. Schiefer. 2016. Normal values for the full visual field, corrected for age and reaction time, using semiautomated kinetic testing on the Octopus 900 perimeter. *Translational Vision Science Technology* 5(2):5.

Groth, S. L., E. F. Linton, E. N. Brown, F. Makadia, and S. P. Donahue. 2023. Evaluation of virtual reality perimetry and standard automated perimetry in normal children. *Translational Vision Science Technology* 12(1):6.

Hashimoto, S., C. Matsumoto, M. Eura, S. Okuyama, and Y. Shimomura. 2017. Evaluation of kinetic programs in various automated perimeters. *Japanese Journal of Ophthalmology* 61:299–306.

Haymes, S. A., D. M. Hutchison, T. A. McCormick, D. K. Varma, M. T. Nicolela., R. P. LeBlanc, and B. C. Chauhan. 2005. Glaucomatous visual field progression with frequency-doubling technology and standard automated perimetry in a longitudinal prospective study. *Investigative Ophthalmology & Visual Science*, 46(2):547–554.

Hepworth, L., and F. Rowe. 2019. Short-listing the program choice for perimetry in neurological conditions (PoPiN) using consensus methods. *The British and Irish Orthoptic Journal* 15(1):125.

Huang, C. Q., J. Carolan, D. Redline, P. Taravati, K. R. Woodward, C. A. Johnson, M. Wall, and J. L. Keltner. 2008. Humphrey matrix perimetry in optic nerve and chiasmal disorders: Comparison with Humphrey SITA standard 24-2. *Investigative Ophthalmology & Visual Science* 49(3):917–923.

Keltner, J. L., C. A. Johnson, J. O. Spurr, and R. W. Beck. 1999. Comparison of central and peripheral visual field properties in the optic neuritis treatment trial. *American Journal of Ophthalmology* 128(5):543–553.

Kumar, A., N. Hekmatjah, Y. Yu, Y. Han, G.-S. Ying, and J. T. Oatts. 2024. Factors associated with visual field testing reliability in children with glaucoma or suspected glaucoma. *American Journal of Ophthalmology* 264:187–193.

Lim, H. W., S. Pershing, D. M. Moshfeghi, H. Heo, M. E. Haque, and S. R. Lambert. 2023. Causes of childhood blindness in the United States using the IRIS® registry (Intelligent Research in Sight). *Ophthalmology* 130(9):907–913.

Ma, X., L. Tang, X. Chen, and L. Zeng. 2021. Periphery kinetic perimetry: Clinically feasible to complement central static perimetry. *BMC Ophthalmology* 21(1):343.

Mees, L., S. Upadhyaya, P. Kumar, S. Kotawala, S. Haran, S. Rajasekar, D. S. Friedman, and R. Venkatesh. 2020. Validation of a head-mounted virtual reality visual field screening device. *Journal of Glaucoma* 29(2):86–91.

Mesfin, Y., A. Kong, B. T. Backus, M. Deiner, Y. Ou, and J. T. Oatts. 2024. Pilot study comparing a new virtual reality-based visual field test to standard perimetry in children. *J AAPOS* 28(3):103933.

Mönter, V. M., D. P. Crabb, and P. H. Artes. 2017. Reclaiming the periphery: Automated kinetic perimetry for measuring peripheral visual fields in patients with glaucoma. *Investigative Ophthalmology & Visual Science* 58(2):868–875.

Morgan, A. M., L. S. Mazzoli, C. Caixeta-Umbelino, and N. Kasahara. 2019. Expediency of the automated perimetry using the Goldmann V stimulus size in visually impaired patients with glaucoma. *Ophthalmology and Therapy* 8(2):305–311.

Narang, P., A. Agarwal, M. Srinivasan, and A. Agarwal. 2021. Advanced vision analyzer-virtual reality perimeter: Device validation, functional correlation and comparison with Humphrey field analyzer. *Ophthalmology Science* 1(2):100035.

Nevalainen, J., J. Paetzold, E. Krapp, R. Vonthein, C. Johnson, and U. Schiefer. 2008. The use of semi-automated kinetic perimetry (SKP) to monitor advanced glaucomatous visual field loss. *Graefe's Archive for Clinical and Experimental Ophthalmology* 246:1331–1339.

Nowomiejska, K., R. Vonthein, J. Paetzold, Z. Zagorski, R. Kardon, and U. Schiefer. 2005. Comparison between semiautomated kinetic perimetry and conventional Goldmann manual kinetic perimetry in advanced visual field loss. *Ophthalmology* 112(8):1343–1354.

Nowomiejska, K., R. Rejdak, Z. Zagorski, and T. Zarnowski. 2009. Comparison of static automated perimetry and semi-automated kinetic perimetry in patients with bilateral visible optic nerve head drusen. *Acta Ophthalmologica* 87(7):801–805.

Nowomiejska, K., R. Vonthein, J. Paetzold, Z. Zagorski, R. Kardon, and U. Schiefer. 2010. Reaction time during semi-automated kinetic perimetry (SKP) in patients with advanced visual field loss. *Acta Ophthalmologica* 88(1):65–69.

Nowomiejska, K., D. Wrobel-Dudzinska, K. Ksiazek, P. Ksiazek, K. Rejdak, R. Maciejewski, A. G. Juenemann, and R. Rejdak. 2015. Semi-automated kinetic perimetry provides additional information to static automated perimetry in the assessment of the remaining visual field in end-stage glaucoma. *Ophthalmic and Physiological Optics* 35(2):147–154.

Oatts, J. T., M. Indaram, and A. G. de Alba Campomanes. 2023. Where have all the pediatric ophthalmologists gone? Pediatric eye care scarcity and the challenge of creating equitable health care access. *JAMA Ophthalmology* 141(3):249–250.

Patel, D. E., P. M. Cumberland, B. C. Walters, I. Russell-Eggitt, M. Cortina-Borja, J. S. Rahi, and OPTIC Study Group. 2015. Study of optimal perimetric testing in children (OPTIC): Feasibility, reliability and repeatability of perimetry in children. *Ophthalmology* 122(8):1711–1717.

Patel, D. E., P. M. Cumberland, B. C. Walters, I. Russell-Eggitt, J. Brookes, M. Papadopoulos, P. T. Khaw, A. C. Viswanathan, D. Garway-Heath, M. Cortina-Borja, J. S. Rahi, and Optimal Perimetric Testing in Children study group. 2018. Comparison of quality and output of different optimal perimetric testing approaches in children with glaucoma. *JAMA Ophthalmology* 136(2):155–161.

Patel, D. E., P. M. Cumberland, B. C. Walters, M. Cortina-Borja, and J. S. Rahi. 2019. Study of optimal perimetric testing in children (OPTIC): Evaluation of kinetic approaches in childhood neuro-ophthalmic disease. *British Journal of Ophthalmology* 103(8):1085–1091.

Phu, J., N. Al-Saleem, M. Kalloniatis, and S. K. Khuu. 2016. Physiologic statokinetic dissociation is eliminated by equating static and kinetic perimetry testing procedures. *Journal of Vision* 16(14):5.

Phu, J., S. K. Khuu, B. Zangerl, and M. Kalloniatis. 2017. A comparison of Goldmann III, V and spatially equated test stimuli in visual field testing: The importance of complete and partial spatial summation. *Ophthalmic and Physiology Optics* 37(2):160–176.

Phu, J., M. Kalloniatis, H. Wang, and S. K. Khuu. 2018. Differences in static and kinetic perimetry results are eliminated in retinal disease when psychophysical procedures are equated. *Translational Vision Science & Technology* 7(5):22.

Phu, J., S. K. Khuu, L. Nivison-Smith, and M. Kalloniatis. 2025. Standard automated perimetry for glaucoma and diseases of the retina and visual pathways: Current and future perspectives. *Progress in Retinal and Eye Research* 104:101307.

Pierre-Filho Pde, T., R. B. Schimiti, J. P. de Vasconcellos, and V. P. Costa. 2006. Sensitivity and specificity of frequency-doubling technology, tendency-oriented perimetry, SITA standard and SITA fast perimetry in perimetrically inexperienced individuals. *Acta Ophthalmology Scandinavica* 84(3):345–350.

Racette, L., M. Fischer, H. Bebie, G. Hollo, C. A. Johnson, and C. Matsumoto. 2019. *Visual field digest: A guide to perimetry and the Octopus perimeter*, 8th ed. https://haag-streit.com/2%20Products/Speciality%20diagnostics/Perimetry/Category%20assets/Books/HS_perimetry_br_xxx_visual_field_digest_8th_en.pdf (accessed February 3, 2025).

Razeghinejad, R., A. Gonzalez-Garcia, J. S. Myers, and L. J. Katz. 2021. Preliminary report on a novel virtual reality perimeter compared with standard automated perimetry. *Journal of Glaucoma* 30(1):17–23.

Rowe, F. J., and A. Rowlands. 2014. Comparison of diagnostic accuracy between Octopus 900 and Goldmann kinetic visual fields. *BioMed Research International* 2014 (1):214829.

Rowe, F. J., C. Noonan, and M. Manuel. 2013. Comparison of Octopus semi-automated kinetic perimetry and Humphrey peripheral static perimetry in neuro-ophthalmic cases. *International Scholarly Research Notices* 2013(1):753202.

Rowe, F. J., C. P. Cheyne, M. García-Fiñana, C. P. Noonan, C. Howard, J. Smith, and J. Adeoye. 2015. Detection of visual field loss in pituitary disease: Peripheral kinetic versus central static. *Neuro-Ophthalmology* 39(3):116–124.

Rowe, F. J., G. Czanner, T. Somerville, I. Sood, and D. Sood. 2021. Octopus 900 automated kinetic perimetry versus standard automated static perimetry in glaucoma practice. *Current Eye Research* 46(1):83–95.

Salt, A., and J. Sargent. 2014. Common visual problems in children with disability. *Archives of Disease in Childhood* 99(12):1163–1168.

Shaarawy, T. M., M. Sherwood, R. Hitchings, and J. Crowston. 2015. *Glaucoma: Medical Diagnosis and Therapy*, vol. 1, 2nd ed. London: Elsevier Limited.

Simpson, M. J. 2017. Mini-review: Far peripheral vision. *Vision Research* 140:96–105.

Sood, D., G. Czanner, T. Somerville, I. Sood, and F. J. Rowe. 2021. Standard automated perimetry using size III and size V stimuli in advanced stage glaucoma: An observational cross-sectional comparative study. *BMJ Open* 11(9):e046124.

Spry, P. G., C. A. Johnson, A. M. McKendrick, and A. Turpin. 2001. Variability components of standard automated perimetry and frequency-doubling technology perimetry. *Investigative Ophthalmology & Visual Science* 42(6):1404–1410.

SSA (U.S. Social Security Administration). n.d. *Disability Evaluation Under Social Security—2.00 Special Senses and Speech—Adult.* https://www.ssa.gov/disability/professionals/bluebook/2.00-SpecialSensesandSpeech-Adult.htm (accessed February 3, 2025).

Stapelfeldt, J., Ş. S. Kucur, N. Huber, R. Höhn, and R. Sznitman. 2021. Virtual reality–based and conventional visual field examination comparison in healthy and glaucoma patients. *Translational Vision Science & Technology* 10(12):10.

Tatham, A. J., F. A. Medeiros, L. M. Zangwill, and R. N. Weinreb. 2015. Strategies to improve early diagnosis in glaucoma. *Progress in Brain Research* 221:103–133. https://doi.org/10.1016/bs.pbr.2015.03.001

Topcon Healthcare. 2025. *Tempo Perimeter.* https://cdn.brandfolder.io/I6S47VV/at/xv4jqq9tgvcnkrkb2fpt9n/TEMPO_Brochure.pdf (accessed February 3, 2025).

Wall, M., R. K. Neahring, and K. R. Woodward. 2002. Sensitivity and specificity of frequency doubling perimetry in neuro-ophthalmic disorders: A comparison with conventional automated perimetry. *Investigative Ophthalmology & Visual Science* 43(4):1277–1283.

Wall, M., C. F. Brito, K. R. Woodward, C. K. Doyle, R. H. Kardon, and C. A. Johnson. 2008. Total deviation probability plots for stimulus size V perimetry: A comparison with size III stimuli. *Archives of Ophthalmology* 126(4):473–479.

Wall, M., C. K. Doyle, K. Zamba, P. Artes, and C. A. Johnson. 2013. The repeatability of mean defect with size III and size V standard automated perimetry. *Investigative Ophthalmology & Visual Science* 54(2):1345–1351.

Wall, M., A. Subramani, L. X. Chong, R. Galindo, A. Turpin, R. H. Kardon, M. J. Thurtell, J. A. Bailey, and I. Marin-Franch. 2019. Threshold static automated perimetry of the full visual field in idiopathic intracranial hypertension. *Investigative Ophthalmology & Visual Science* 60(6):1898–1905.

Walsh, H. L., A. Parrish, L. Hucko, J. Sridhar, and K. M. Cavuoto. 2023. Access to pediatric ophthalmological care by geographic distribution and US population demographic characteristics in 2022. *JAMA Ophthalmology* 141(3):242–249.

Wang, B., S. Alvarez-Falcón, M. El-Dairi, and S. F. Freedman. 2023. Performance of virtual reality game-based automated perimetry in patients with childhood glaucoma. *Journal of American Association for Pediatric Ophthalmology and Strabismus* 27(6):325.e1–325.e6.

Wilscher, S., B. Wabbels, and B. Lorenz. 2010. Feasibility and outcome of automated kinetic perimetry in children. *Graefe's Archive for Clinical and Experimental Ophthalmology* 248:1493–1500.

Wroblewski, D., B. A. Francis, A. Sadun, G. Vakili, and V. Chopra. 2014. Testing of visual field with virtual reality goggles in manual and visual grasp modes. *BioMed Research International* 2014:206082.

Yohannan, J., J. Wang, J. Brown, B. C. Chauhan, M. V. Boland, D. S. Friedman, and P. Y. Ramulu. 2017. Evidence-based criteria for assessment of visual field reliability. *Ophthalmology* 124(11):1612–1620.

Yoon, M. K., T. N. Hwang, S. Day, J. Hong, T. Porco, and T. J. McCulley. 2012. Comparison of Humphrey matrix frequency doubling technology to standard automated perimetry in neuro-ophthalmic disease. *Middle East African Journal of Ophthalmology* 19(2):211–215.

Appendix A

Public Meeting Agendas

COMMITTEE ON REVIEW OF STANDARDS FOR VISUAL FIELD PERIMETRY DEVICES AND THEIR USE IN DISABILITY EVALUATIONS

Virtual Public Session

SEPTEMBER 20, 2024

12:30–12:40	**Welcome and Introductions** Roger Lewis, *Committee Chair*
12:40–1:00	**Social Security Administration Overview** Vince Nibali, *Technical Expert,* Office of Medical Policy, Social Security Administration
1:00–1:45	**Questions and Discussion** Committee Members and SSA Staff
1:45	**Adjourn Public Session**

COMMITTEE ON REVIEW OF STANDARDS FOR VISUAL FIELD PERIMETRY DEVICES AND THEIR USE IN DISABILITY EVALUATIONS

Virtual Public Session

OCTOBER 30, 2024

9:10–9:15 Welcome and Introductions
Roger Lewis, *Committee Chair*

9:15–10:15 Session I: Disparities and Opportunities in Access to Vision Testing
Robert Chun, *Committee Member*

Panelist Remarks
Varshini Varadaraj, Johns Hopkins Disability Health Center
Yao Liu, University of Wisconsin–Madison
Paula Anne Newman-Casey, University of Michigan Kellogg Eye Center

Q&A with Panelists

10:15–11:00 Session II: Challenges in Access to Vision Testing—Lived Experiences
Eve Higgenbotham, *Committee Member*

Q&A with Panelists
Christopher Hord, Washington
LaQuilla Harris, Maryland
Zelda Kitchens, Alabama

11:00–11:15 Break

11:15–12:30 Session III: Emerging Technologies in Visual Field Testing
Stuart Gardiner, *Committee Member*

Panelist Remarks
Chris Johnson, University of Iowa
Sylvia Groth, Vanderbilt University
George Spaeth, Wills Eye Hospital

Q&A with Panelists

12:30 Adjourn Public Session

Appendix B

Glossary

Algorithm: See *perimetric algorithm*.
Apostilb: A unit of luminance referred to in the SSA listings.
Applicability: The extent to which the results of a perimetry technique can be generalized to the target population and setting for which the test is intended. In other words, it assesses whether the study's findings are relevant and applicable to the specific clinical context in which the test is meant to be used.
Automated (or automatic) kinetic perimetry: See *semiautomated kinetic perimetry*, a term used preferentially in this report to better reflect the role of the technician operating the test.
Automated perimetry: Automated presentation of the test stimulus and recording of patient responses (EyeWiki, 2024).
Blind spot: An area of the visual field in which a stimulus is not seen at any intensity.
Bowl perimeter (or bowl perimetry device): A perimetry device wherein an examinee looks into a bowl-shaped surface, upon which stimuli are projected. Includes most common perimeters used today, such as the Humphrey Field Analyzer and Octopus lines of products, as well as the original Goldmann perimeter.
Candela: The International System of Units (SI) unit of luminance. Referred to in the SSA listings.
Cecocentral area: The area of the visual field from the physiologic blind spot (approximately 15 degrees temporal to fixation) to central fixation (Araie et al., 1995).

Confrontation test: An examination in which a clinician moves their finger(s) in and out of the examinee's field of view and asks when they can see and/or count the finger(s).

Contrast sensitivity: The minimum stimulus intensity (brightness) that a patient can detect at a specific location within the visual field, expressed in decibels (dB) on visual fields. Higher dB values indicate better function (i.e., detection of a dimmer stimulus) on visual field results.

Decibels (dB): "A measure of attenuation, where a higher dB score indicates the ability to perceive a stimulus of lower intensity (i.e., greater contrast sensitivity)" (Phu et al., 2025).

Defect severity: The degree to which an area of the visual field has lower contrast sensitivity than expected (Patel et al., 2007).

False-negative response: An indication that an examinee does not see a stimulus where one is present that the examinee would be expected to detect easily.

False-positive response: An indication that an examinee reports seeing a stimulus where one is not present.

Fixation loss: When an examinee's gaze deviates from the fixation point during a perimetric exam.

Fixation point: A designated spot upon which a perimetric examinee is told to maintain their gaze.

Frequency doubling technology (FDT): A perimetric technology based on a flicker illusion, which essentially creates an image that appears double its actual spatial frequency. Although the stimulus does not move across the field, the flickering is a proxy for the stimulus intensity used in either static or kinetic perimetry (EyeWiki, 2023).

Goldmann stimulus size: A standard size scale for circular perimetric stimuli. The sizes, numbered I–V, each cover four times the area of the previous size.

Hill of vision: A term referring to a three-dimensional representation of the visual field, where the peak of the "hill" corresponds to the fovea (the point of highest visual sensitivity), and where the sensitivity gradually decreases away from the center of vision towards the periphery, creating a slope similar to a hill's terrain.

Humphrey Field Analyzer (HFA): The primary perimeter used in the United States. The HFA is an automated static threshold perimeter.

Kinetic perimetry: A method of visual field testing using a moving stimulus where the stimulus is generally moved from a nonseeing area to a seeing area in a systematic way to map the central and peripheral visual field boundaries, in addition to any scotomas, including blind spots. This movement can be automated, semiautomated, or manual.

Luminance: The brightness of an object presented to the eye; perimetry devices report the maximum luminance of a stimulus and the background luminance (Phu et al., 2025).

APPENDIX B										135

Mean deviation or mean defect (MD): The average difference in visual field sensitivity across all measured locations, compared to a normal, age-matched reference field.

Meridians: Imaginary lines that divide the visual field into equal sections, like pieces of a pie. Typically, the visual field is divided into eight equal sections, with the meridians radiating out from the central focus point. These radii are labeled in degrees moving counterclockwise from the 3 o'clock position (0, 45, 90, 135, 180, 225, 270, and 315 degrees for an eight-meridian scheme). The radii may also be labeled using anatomical references: nasally (0 degrees in the left eye and 180 degrees in the right eye), up nasally, superiorly (90 degrees in both eyes), up temporally, temporally (180 degrees in the left eye and 0 degrees in the right eye), down temporally, inferiorly (270 degrees in both eyes), and down nasally (IMAIOS, n.d.).

Optical projection: Perimetry performed by projecting a light stimulus onto a background to present it to the patient's eye in order to map the visual field.

Perimeter: A machine used to measure visual fields.

Perimetric algorithm: A statistical package that comes onboard with perimetric hardware and is used to mathematically estimate the boundaries of an examinee's visual field. Generally independent of an individual's results from prior testing sessions.

Perimetry: See *visual perimetry*.

Physiologic blind spot: The area where there is expected to be no visual sensitivity, corresponding to the location of the optic nerve.

Reliability indices: Indicators of the confidence with which one can ascertain whether the results of a single test are credible or if they require repetition or rejection.

Reproducibility: Also referred to in the literature as "reliability," but for the purposes of this report, reproducibility is the degree to which results remain consistent (or are less variable) over repeated measurements.

Scotoma: An area that falls within the boundary of the visual field in which stimuli are not seen at an intensity expected in that location.

Semiautomated kinetic perimetry: A visual field test that uses a moving stimulus of a selected size and intensity, with the speed and direction of the stimulus being automated.

Sensitivity: In the context of this report, a test's ability to correctly identify those with a qualifying disability. (Not to be confused with "contrast sensitivity" defined above.)

Specificity: In the context of this report, a test's ability to correctly identify those without a qualifying disability.

Static perimetry: A visual field test during which stationary stimuli are presented at defined points in the visual field. Locations at which the stimulus is seen and not seen are recorded.

Static automated threshold perimetry (static or standard automated perimetry (SAP), "white on white" perimetry): Visual field test that uses the projection of a white stimulus onto a white background to determine the probable threshold at chosen locations in the visual field. Blue on yellow static automated threshold perimetry is also available.

Statutory blindness, federal definition: "Central visual acuity of 20/200 or less in the better eye with the use of correcting lens. An eye which has a limitation in the field of vision so that the widest diameter of the visual field subtends an angle no greater than 20 degrees is considered to have a central visual acuity of 20/200 or less."[1]

Subthreshold (stimulus): A stimulus below the estimated detection threshold of a normal visual field location.

Suprathreshold (stimulus): A stimulus "above the estimated detection threshold of a normal visual field location" (Artes et al., 2003).

Tangent screen test: A manual method of assessing the central and peripheral visual field using a flat black screen (usually 1 to 2 meters away) and a moving target. It is useful for detecting functional vision loss, neurologic field defects, and scotomas.

Threshold: The stimulus intensity that a person can detect on 50 percent of presentations.

Threshold testing: Perimetric examination that calculates the precise contrast sensitivity of various locations in the eye.

Validity: The ability of a perimetry technique to accurately identify whether an individual meets the criteria for disability.

Visual acuity: A measure of the sharpness or clarity of vision at a given distance where normal vision is 20/20 (CHOP, n.d.).

Visual acuity efficiency, SSA definition: "A percentage that corresponds to the best-corrected central visual acuity for distance in [the] better eye" (SSA, n.d.). It is based on a reference chart that aligns Snellen visual acuity metrics with visual acuity efficiency percentages.

Visual acuity impairment value, SSA definition: "Corresponds to the best-corrected central visual acuity for distance in [the] better eye" (SSA, n.d.). It is based on a reference chart using Snellen metrics.

Visual efficiency, SSA definition: "A calculated value of [the] remaining visual function, [combining the] visual acuity efficiency and [the] visual field efficiency[, expressed] as a percentage" (SSA, n.d.). For example, if the visual acuity efficiency percentage is 75 and the visual field efficiency percentage is 40, the visual efficiency percentage is (75 × 40) / 100 = 30 percent.

Visual field: The total area in which objects can be seen by either or both eyes while focusing on a central point; the right visual field is perceived by the right eye and the left visual field is perceived by the left eye.

---

[1] § 404.1581

Visual field includes both central vision and peripheral vision, which is the ability to see objects to the side or up and down while looking straight ahead (Medline Plus, 2023).

Visual field efficiency, SSA definition: "A percentage that corresponds to the visual field in [the] better eye. ... the visual field efficiency percentage [is calculated] by adding the number of degrees [seen] along the eight principal meridians found on a visual field chart (0, 45, 90, 135, 180, 225, 270, 315) in your better eye and dividing by 5" (SSA, n.d.). For example, if the visual field is contracted down to 25 degrees in all eight meridians, the remaining visual field efficiency would be (25 × 8) / 5 = 40 percent.

Visual field impairment value, SSA definition: "Corresponds to the visual field in [the] better eye. Using the [mean deviation (MD)] from acceptable automated static threshold perimetry, [SSA calculates] the visual field impairment value by dividing the absolute value of the MD by 22" (SSA, n.d.).

Visual field index: A "global metric that represents the entire visual field as a single number. It is estimated by calculating age corrected defect depth at the test points identified as significantly depressed in pattern deviation probability maps" (Iutaka et al., 2017).

Visual impairment value, SSA definition: "A calculated value of [a person's] loss of visual function, [combining the] visual acuity impairment value and [the] visual field impairment value" (SSA, n.d.).

Visual perimeter device: See *perimeter*.

Visual perimetry: Systemic measurement of the visual field.

REFERENCES

Araie, M., M. Arai, N. Koseki, and Y. Suzuki. 1995. Influence of myopic refraction on visual field defects in normal tension and primary open angle glaucoma. *Japanese Journal of Ophthalmology* 39(1):60–64.

Artes, P. H., D. B. Henson, R. Harper, and D. McLeod. 2003. Multisampling suprathreshold perimetry: A comparison with conventional suprathreshold and full-threshold strategies by computer simulation. *Investigative Ophthalmology & Visual Science* 44(6):2582–2587.

CHOP (Children's Hospital of Philadelphia). n.d. *Functional Vision.* https://www.chop.edu/conditions-diseases/functional-vision (accessed February 4, 2025).

EyeWiki. 2023. *Frequency doubling technology.* https://eyewiki.org/Frequency_Doubling_Technology (accessed January 29, 2025).

EyeWiki. 2024. *Standard automated perimetry.* https://eyewiki.org/Standard_Automated_Perimetry#Manual_vs._Automated_Perimetry (accessed January 29, 2025).

IMAIOS. n.d. *Meridians of eyeball.* https://www.imaios.com/en/e-anatomy/anatomical-structures/meridians-of-eyeball-1557868088 (accessed February 7, 2025).

Iutaka, N. A., R. A. Grochowski, and N. Kasahara. 2017. Correlation between visual field index and other functional and structural measures in glaucoma patients and suspects. *Journal of Ophthalmic and Vision Research* 12(1):53–57.

Medline Plus. 2023. *Visual field.* https://medlineplus.gov/ency/article/003879.htm (accessed January 29, 2025).

Patel, A., G. Wollstein, H. Ishikawa, and J. S. Schuman. 2007. Comparison of visual field defects using matrix perimetry and standard achromatic perimetry. *Ophthalmology* 114(3):480–487.

Phu, J., S. K. Khuu, L. Nivison-Smith, and M. Kalloniatis. 2025. Standard automated perimetry for glaucoma and diseases of the retina and visual pathways: Current and future perspectives. *Progress in Retinal and Eye Research* 104:101307.

SSA (U.S. Social Security Administration). n.d. *Disability evaluation under Social Security—2.00 Special senses and speech—Adult.* https://www.ssa.gov/disability/professionals/bluebook/2.00-SpecialSensesandSpeech-Adult.htm (accessed February 4, 2025).

Appendix C

Biographical Sketches of Committee Members

Roger Lewis, M.D., Ph. D (*Chair*), is a professor of emergency medicine at the David Geffen School of Medicine at the University of California, Los Angeles, and a senior medical scientist at Berry Consultants, LLC, a group that specializes in innovative clinical trial design. Dr. Lewis is the senior statistical editor for *JAMA* and editor of the *JAMA* series entitled "JAMA Guides to Statistics and Methods." His expertise centers on adaptive and Bayesian clinical trials, including platform trials; general clinical research methodology; data and safety monitoring boards; and the oversight of clinical trials. Dr. Lewis was formerly the chair of the Department of Emergency Medicine at Harbor–UCLA Medical Center and a senior physician in the Los Angeles County Department of Health Services. He has authored or coauthored more than 270 original research publications, reviews, editorials, and chapters. Dr. Lewis is a past president of the Society for Academic Emergency Medicine and served on the board of directors for the Society for Clinical Trials. He is a fellow of the American Statistical Association and the Society for Clinical Trials. Dr. Lewis is an active member of the National Academy of Medicine.

Robert Chun, OD, is an associate clinical professor at the State University of New York College of Optometry. He has been a low vision specialist and clinician educator since 2012. Dr. Chun has been devoted to understanding the functional aspects of vision loss experienced by those affected by retinitis pigmentosa and Stargardt disease. Currently, his studies seek to advance our understanding of how and when various aspects of functional endpoints are affected by disease progression among those living with low vision.

Dr. Chun has served as a coinvestigator and collaborator in National Eye Institute–funded studies involving low-vision technologies. He is a fellow of the American Academy of Optometry. Outside of teaching in the classroom, clinic, and research laboratory, Dr. Chun has extensive experience working with visually impaired athletes through his role as a vision impairment classifier for the International Paralympic Committee.

Stuart Gardiner, Ph.D., is a senior scientist at Devers Eye Institute in Portland, Oregon. His primary research involves developing, evaluating, and learning from advances in diagnostic testing for glaucoma for the purposes of disease detection, assessing and predicting the rate of disease progression, and uncovering the underlying pathophysiological processes. In particular, Dr. Gardiner has focused on functional testing of the visual field using automated perimetry; blood flow within the retina and optic nerve; and structural evaluation of the optic nerve head. He has been continuously funded as a principal investigator by the National Eye Institute since 2011, with grants related to functional testing and retinal blood flow. Dr. Gardiner is a gold fellow of the Association for Research in Vision and Ophthalmology. He served as an advisor to Haag Streit at a one-time meeting in July 2024 and received compensation for those services.

Eve Higginbotham, SM, M.D., ML, is a professor of ophthalmology and senior fellow at the Leonard Davis Institute for Health Economics. She has also served for a decade (2013–2024) as the inaugural vice dean for inclusion, diversity, and equity at the University of Pennsylvania. Dr. Higginbotham continues to publish on topics in the fields of ophthalmology, organizational culture, health policy, and health equity. She is an elected and active member of the National Academy of Medicine (NAM), and she recently completed a six-year term (2018–2024) as a member of the NAM council. During this time, she chaired the NAM finance committee and served on the National Research Council and as NAM liaison to the National Academy of Sciences investment committee. A glaucoma specialist, Dr. Higginbotham holds degrees in chemical engineering, medicine, and law.

Tianjing Li, Ph.D., is a professor of ophthalmology and epidemiology at University of Colorado Anschutz Medical Campus. The primary focus of Dr. Li's research is to develop, evaluate, and disseminate rigorous methods for comparing health care interventions and to provide trustworthy evidence for decision making. She has garnered an international reputation as a leader in comparative effectiveness research (clinical trials, systematic review, network meta-analysis) and patient-centered outcomes research.

Dr. Li has extensive experience in applying these methods in ophthalmology and optometry. She serves as a coeditor-in-chief for the journal *Trials*; a methodological editor for *Annals of Internal Medicine*; the reviews editor for *JAMA Ophthalmology*; an associate scientific editor for the second edition of the *Cochrane Handbook for Systematic Reviews of Interventions*; a section editor for the book *Principles and Practice of Clinical Trials*; and is author and editor for the second edition of the *Textbook of Epidemiology*. Dr. Li is an elected fellow of the Society for Research Synthesis Methodology and served as the society's president from 2022 to 2023. She has served on two previous National Academies of Sciences, Engineering, and Medicine committees.

Julius Oatts, M.D., is an associate professor at the Children's Hospital of Philadelphia and the University of Pennsylvania School of Medicine. Previously, he created and led the childhood glaucoma clinic at the University of California, San Francisco. Dr. Oatts has clinical expertise in the medical and surgical management of childhood glaucoma. His research expertise includes childhood vision screening for preventable vision loss and evaluating new diagnostic technologies in pediatric ophthalmology. Dr. Oatts is a member of the American Association of Pediatric Ophthalmology and Strabismus (AAPOS), the American Glaucoma Society, the American Academy of Ophthalmology, and the North American Pediatric Glaucoma Society. He serves as vice chair of the AAPOS professional education committee and technology committee.

Eric Singman, M.D., is a professor of ophthalmology and visual sciences and a professor of neurology at the University of Maryland (UMD) School of Medicine. He is a board-certified ophthalmologist with fellowship training in neuro-ophthalmology. Before joining UMD, Dr. Singman founded and directed the Wilmer Clinic for Vision Concerns after Traumatic Brain Injury and cofounded the Wilmer Genetic Eye Disease Center at The Johns Hopkins Hospital. His research interests have focused on optimization of delivery of eye care, the impact of brain injury on vision, and the visual sequelae of Ehler's Danlos syndrome. Dr. Singman served on the medical advisory panel of BravoVictor (the blind veterans' foundation for both the United Kingdom and United States) from 2022 to 2024. He also consults as a district medical adviser for the U.S. Department of Labor Federal Occupational Health in evaluating visual system disability claim reports for federal employees with work-related injuries. Dr. Singman is a fellow of the Royal Society of Medicine of the United Kingdom and a member of the North American Neuro-ophthalmology Society, the American Academy of Ophthalmology, and the American Military Surgeons of the United States.